KEEP THE
FIRES
BURNING

Conquering stress and burnout as a Mother-Baby Professional

Micky Jones, BS, CLD, CD(DONA), HCHI, IBCLC, DFB

Keep the Fires Burning: Conquering Stress and Burnout as a Mother-Baby Professional

Micky Jones, BS, CLD, CD(DONA), HCHI, IBCLC, DFB

Praeclarus Press, LLC

2504 Sweetgum Lane

Amarillo, Texas 79124 USA

806-367-9950

www.PraeclarusPress.com

DISCLAIMER

The information contained in this publication is advisory only and is not intended to replace sound clinical judgment or individualized patient care. The author disclaims all warranties, whether expressed or implied, including any warranty as the quality, accuracy, safety, or suitability of this information for any particular purpose.

ISBN: 978-1-939807-73-1

Endorsements

The prevention of "burn out" is an important and timely topic. Micky Jones has given us a heartfelt, sensible guide that will become a very necessary addition to every doula library, as well as all midwifery and doula education programs.

Barbara Harper, RN, CLD, CCCE, DEM
Founder - Waterbirth International
Author - *Gentle Birth Choices*
Creator - Waterbirth Certification & Gentle Birth Guardian Workshops
CAPPA Labor Doula Trainer

Timing is everything - and there couldn't be a more timely work than Micky's book on birth worker burnout. I have been kidding around with this issue for a while; "Ha! I need an intervention" or "I'm a birth junkie, ho, ho, ho!" and so on, as if it were funny. But, sadly, it's not funny. Not at all. We all take our work seriously; often times it can be a matter of life and death. Dedication to the greater cause drives us all, but I, for one, am thankful for some guidance along the way. Literally, in the nick of time, I received the gift of this book from Micky. Two words - 'self care' - had recently found their way into my vocabulary as I had begun to spin out of control. I found solace in these pages as Micky outlined the steps to implementing a sensible, doable plan to establish 'self care.' You can do it, too - you know it's long overdue. Take care of yourself, so you can keep taking care of others. ***Congrats Micky, and thank you!***

Jennie Joseph LM, CPM Midwife
Executive Director - Commonsense Childbirth Inc./ The Birth Place
Founder of 'The JJ Way'

Micky Jones has dared confront the decidedly un-lovely side of being a mother-baby professional. By doing so, she allows us to face the aspects of our work that can lead to burnout, and more importantly, what we can do about them. She poignantly describes her own journey through burnout, promising us that on the other side of that difficult experience, we'll find joy. *Keep the Fires Burning* is a delightfully well-written and practical guide for anyone who works with mothers and babies. Let your self-care journey begin here. You'll be glad you did.

Kathleen Kendall-Tackett, Ph.D., IBCLC, FAPA

Author, *The Hidden Feelings of Motherhood and Depression in New Mothers*

Dedication

This book is dedicated to my family:

To my children for teaching me about motherhood and giving me my life's work.

To my husband for deciding that it is easier just to love me.

I love you.

Acknowledgments

There are so many people I could thank and recognize as supporters through this process. Writing a book was much harder than I ever thought it would be. I have always had a lot to say, as the comments on my 2nd grade report card pointed out, yet writing them down in a coherent manner proved more challenging than I had ever dreamed. I am so thankful that I can put a stake at the top of this mountain and declare it accomplished.

Thank you to Kathy Kendall-Tackett, my editor when this journey began, and the person who spent many conversations at conferences, during phone calls, and through emails encouraging me to quit making outlines and just write something. Without your encouragement, I would not have taken a step down this path. Thank you for believing in me and for talking sense into me many times. You are one of my heroes and I am honored to call you a friend.

Thank you to Thomas Hale and the Hale Publishing crew for your support. You are helping me make my dreams come true.

I have many mentors and sisters in the cause who have poured into my life professionally and personally. Jennie Joseph, Barbara Harper, Barbara Nicholson, Lyssa Parker, Kerry Tuschoff, Kim Durdin, Teresa Howard, Michelle-Nicholle Calareso, and Mary Anne Richardson – thank you for your love, prayers, and belief in me. I love you.

I am blessed with a life full of wonderful people, but hold only a few as close friends. Thanks to Jessie Hawkins and my entire GCM crew for loving me, even when I wasn't around. Caroline Andrews – thanks for being my Zumba® hip scarf twin and so much more. Thanks girls for being my friends and sisters.

To my 9 Months & Beyond, LLC team and family I extend my deepest gratitude. Thank you for your support as I ditched you for several months in order to spend days sequestered away writing. I am so glad we support each other when we need to take a break or do something crazy like write a book. Sarah & Bryan McKay, Kate Cropp, Libby and the crew – thank you for being my family.

Of course without my own trip down a path of stress and a road up towards recovery, I would not have this story to tell. Thankfully, my therapist, Alice Strickland and the Refuge Center in Franklin, TN, were there to support and guide me. I am grateful to you for sharing your skills and compassion with the world. Thanks also to Dani Williamson, my nurse practitioner, and the staff at Cool Springs Family Medicine whose dedication to truly holistic health has put me back on the path of health and wellness.

Thank you to all the mother-baby professionals, friends, family, and acquaintances on Twitter, Facebook, message boards, and "real life" that encouraged me to write, saying this book would help lots of people. I sure hope you are right! For those who shared stories, filled out surveys, and were happy to help – thank you for sharing and lending your voice to help someone else.

My Four Winds Mission/ Windfarm Cafe family is my rock of love and belonging. Thank you for teaching me valuable lessons about vulnerability and joy. Even though our journey is just beginning, I am so blessed to walk with you. Thank you for your support during this process.

Finally, thank you to my wonderful family. To my excited parents (and step parents) who can't wait to read a book that has nothing to do with them, but happens to be written by their baby, thank you for never giving up on our relationship, despite the difficult times. I am so thankful to my giving, supportive mother-in-law Brenda Marshall for all your amazing contributions. I could not have written this book without you.

My husband, K.C. Jones, and my children, Abigayle, Ambrose, and Paul – you are my joy and the light that illuminated the way down the path of caring for mothers and babies. Without you I would not have my passion. KC, thank you for supporting my "writing retreats" and for the greatest, calmest tech support ever during the great computer debacles. Thank you all for your love all along the way, even when I was lost and confused. You are my greatest gifts. I love you.

Soli Deo Gloria

Foreword

For many people in today's society, stress is a chronic and recurrent problem, and its costs, when undetected or untreated, are enormous. One group, in particular, is the audience for this enlightened book into which Micky Jones has poured her heart, soul, and mind. She has skillfully addressed the unique dilemmas that come with being a mother-baby professional. The path she lays before us of help and healing that anyone, not just birth professionals, can follow, can lead the reader to understanding and possibly preventing burnout in their own lives.

With refreshing clarity and insight, Micky Jones has us look at the realities of providing care for pregnant, birthing, and postpartum women as a doula, lactation consultant, or midwife. Whether they practice within the medical establishment of hospitals or outside the security oriented mind-set of modern medicine, each mother-baby profession has its own set of challenges to the women (and men) that choose to work with families during the birth year.

Jones claims too many eager doulas begin a practice only to find that the realities of life on call 24/7, the urge to always be there for their clients, combined with family obligations and the necessity to actually build a business from this hands-on calling, cause many mother-baby professionals (MBPs) to leave after only a few years. This book gives us concrete evidence of the consequences–physically, mentally, and emotionally, of the professional tendency to put clients' and family needs before individual needs.

Laid out in an easy-to-follow sequence, this book helps the reader recognize their own ways of practicing, their methods of coping, and how each professional might want to adjust their perspective to prevent waking up one day and not wanting to do this work anymore. On a very practical level, what Micky Jones has done is give us a basic prescription for success in this field, rather than a prevention for burnout. Because along with the mindfulness that she so deftly creates in her "basics" strategy, she is giving each person the encouragement they need to be the best possible person. And when you develop character and integrity by caring for your own needs, then you can easily become the best possible mother-baby professional, wife, partner, mother, sister, or friend.

If the well researched discourse on the causes and cures of stress in our lives is the mind of this book, then its heart is Micky's personal story of looking into the mirror and taking stock of her own life as a busy, self proclaimed overachiever, and mother who just wanted the merry-go-round to stop for a few days. I won't reveal her tender and moving account of how she took matters into her own hands, but will tell you that it was very similar to my own story, as just a year before Micky faced her mirror I looked into mine.

I am a mother-baby professional who has stood the test of time, having been working in the healthcare field for 40 years. Yes, there were days when I wanted to give up working against the current of medicalized birth, but something always kept me going until January 3, 2008. That was my day of looking into the mirror and contemplating not just quitting, but doing something more drastic. Similar to the tapestry Micky Jones weaves of her life out of balance, I was overcommitted physically and emotionally and undernourished spiritually. Many things saved me that year, but the most important, I believe, was connecting to God on a deep, personal, and emotional level. Plus I turned off all distractions to spending time alone with spiritual teachings–no TV, radio, newspapers, or even music. I finally could hear myself and what was needed to survive. I simply stopped and the world didn't end. It got easier and easier to say "no" because each time I said it I was saying "yes" to myself. I started eating simply, exercising (which was a big deal for someone who was morbidly obese and morbidly afraid of sweat), and spending more time with family and friends. It took over a year to drop 100 pounds and that was the insignificant part of the year. The most significant part was that I created a new way of seeing myself that resonated with every fiber of my being. Dropping the weight was incidental to connecting on a deeper level.

As I read through this amazingly simple, yet powerful book, I kept thinking to myself, "I wish I had had this about three years, or even ten years, before my collapse." This book would have awakened me, given me direction, encouraged me to connect, and helped me see that I was not breaking down, but breaking out. Micky Jones gently and lovingly helps those who love to help others see the wisdom of "healing the healer." I created a workshop in 1982, as a member of the Board of Directors of the American Holistic Nurses Association, to address the problems that nurses' encounter in working such fast-paced, demanding jobs. The workshops were successful and used some of the simple guidance that is contained in this book. But the research Micky brings to light and the depth that she illuminates its impact on our lives has completely surpassed what I was doing in the early 80s.

I feel confident that "Keep the Fires Burning" will help mother-baby professionals, as well as student midwives, beginning doulas, and even their young daughters take a good look at their lives from many different perspectives. Living a life in balance is not an easy accomplishment in today's emailing, texting, and twittering world, but Micky Jones has passed on a legacy to all those who are ready to do a better job for themselves, their families, and ultimately the women they are so eager to serve.

Barbara Harper, RN, CLD, CCCE, Midwife
Author *Gentle Birth Choices*
Director Waterbirth International

Table of Contents

Introduction

Twinkle, Twinkle Little Star
How I wonder what you are

> *Up above the world so high*
> *Like a diamond in the sky*

> > *Twinkle, Twinkle Little Star*
> > *How I wonder what you are*

> > -Traditional children's song

You're through. Finished. Burned out. Used up. You've been
replaced...forgotten. That's a lie!

> - Charles R. Swindoll

Labor Doula, Postpartum Doula, Lactation Consultant, Childbirth Educator, Midwife. Perhaps you have one of these titles or a combination of two, three, or more. Or perhaps you have another name that describes the work you do assisting families as they usher new human beings earth-side and learn to nurture them. The term I have come to use for those of us who work with mothers and their babies and the term I will use throughout this book is *mother-baby professional (MBP)*. This is someone who is not typically a medical professional (but could be a doctor, nurse, or, of course, midwife), but is an allied health professional who supports women and their infants in the perinatal period. I do, however, include midwives in this group, even though many categorize them as medical professionals. Midwives can also suffer from the same stress and burnout as other mother-baby professionals due to the level of emotional intensity, uncertainty, and political juggling that comes with the midwifery model of care, especially in the United States. These women (and some men) might also be called "birth workers." MBPs are people who fill the roles that were once filled by family, friends, and community members. Our "professional ancestors" are the other women who came to support a mother during her labor–the wise woman in the community who could get a baby to latch just right, the traditional midwife, like my own great grandmother, who caught all the babies in her small, Black Muslim community. Those women established our collective legacy and represent the gap we aim to fill. Essentially, as a mother-baby professional, you carry on the wise woman[1] tradition as an advocate for mothers and babies–a passionate servant and guide, helping families as they journey through the delicate years of childbearing and early parenthood.

As a mother-baby professional that wears many hats, it has become an easier way to refer to myself versus always explaining how to pronounce D-O-U-L-A, then explain what it is, *and then* launch into all the other mother-baby related certifications I hold. As I have had the pleasure of training, working with, and getting to know many doulas, lactation consultants, childbirth educators, midwives, etc. over the years, the same conversation always creeps up. It starts off as a joke or two about needing toothpicks to hold up the eyelids or a familiar story of being disrespected by a doctor who didn't get "all the fuss about breastfeeding." We joke, we tell each other stories, and we respond with that knowing glance and a sympathetic nod. But it's not really all that funny. What does it matter if more and more women are dedicating their lives to helping other women with the childbearing years if they only last for a few years before calling it quits? We live on coffee and chocolate, just hoping to make it through another day. We preach, "Take care of yourself!" to new parents, while suffering from stress-induced illness and disease ourselves! Too many of us are tired or sick, or just plain sick and tired–suffering from emotional stress, physical stress, and eventually burnout.

Thinking about these conversations with other passionate mother-baby professionals made me wonder if a high level of stress was just an inherent part of working with pregnant and newly parenting families or if it could be minimized. Maybe it could even be avoided by structuring work or professional life in a specific way. Was there some secret to having a thriving practice, a healthy family, and glowing inner-peace? I was certainly interested in the answer and I figured many others who loved working with mothers and babies would want to know the answer, too. This has been my meandering quest to find out that secret. Can life as a mother-baby professional be interesting, fulfilling, passionate, and free of burnout? I don't know that I uncovered a miraculous secret, but I did discover strategies that will change your career and life for the better if you are brave enough to take an honest look at your current situation and make changes in your life. Changes that can bring you more fulfillment by helping you live a more authentic, lower stress life.

My hope is that you are reading this as a happy, healthy professional, looking

---

1   For ease, throughout this book I will refer to MBPs as mothers/women/her, as the majority of us in this field are women. The information on stress and developing a personal care plan are applicable to either gender. If you are a male doula, lactation consultant, or midwife, you are already used to the feminine, so I know you can handle it.

for information to stay low-stress and prevent long-term burnout. But as a woman with an uncanny ability to ignore the bright side, I realize it's more likely you picked up this book because you are struggling. You are already stressed to the max, wondering how long you can hold up before you pack up all your technical books and supplies and get a job where you can clock in and out and just be done when the day is over. I know–I lived in that weird place of wondering if you will ever love what you do again. You may be done with this work. You know you want to pack it up, but want to leave with a feeling of closure. Perhaps your answer will be a restructuring of how you serve mothers and babies. And perhaps you will find making a clear plan to release stress and combat burnout will allow you to enjoy a long career doing just what you do now. Whatever your path, I hope my journey and collection of wisdom gives some light and hope.

I've written this book in three parts to give you the background information you need or desire, and to help you start making a self-care plan right away. The first is a brief overview of stress as it relates specifically to MBPs and generally to members of Western culture. The second segment is a simple exploration of stress in its many forms, so you might recognize it as it appears in your life. Third, and perhaps the most important segment is dedicated to developing a personal self-care plan to help you live a happier, healthier, low stress life! A list of resources is in the back for additional reading. Unfortunately, stress and burnout are at such epidemic levels in our society that I could read a new book on stress each month and never run out of reading material. I have included those that have been a part of my journey and I know will be helpful on yours.

Chapter 1

What Are Things Like Out There?

Frustration, stress, and burnout are common topics of conversation among mother-baby professionals. Feeling overwhelmed and becoming increasingly frustrated, thousands of doulas, childbirth educators, and midwives leave the mother-baby field each year (Antunes, 2009). Antunes (2009) refers to this feeling as the "Three-Year Itch," while others describe it as stress, feeling worn-out, or life just feeling wrong. Whatever you call it, bright stars in our field are burning out—either changing careers or leaving the field all together.

> *I've been involved with a group doula practice for the past 10 years. I took over running the practice two years ago. Over the past ten years, I've seen almost all the doulas that were originally involved stop practice. I've also seen many doulas join us, hang around for a few years, then leave the field.*
>
> -Angela Horn, CD(DONA), CCCE, CBC, CHBE, CPD
> (ten years in mother-baby field)

> *Some of the stress for me is working with employers who do not appreciate and value the services provided by me. So most of my stress level, which I generally feel is high, is based on working with the employer, not with the patients.*
>
> -D.J., IBCLC (22 years in lactation)

> *The advocacy aspect of my job as a doula leaves me worn-out. I routinely see interventions that are not life-saving and that mothers don't really want or need, but that they consent to while in labor out of fear...because as a doula I can't speak for them or tell them what to do, I simply bear witness to births that are more traumatic and rushed than they need to be. That is so hard when I know it can be different. Caregivers also routinely lie or manipulate to get women to do what they want, and I am pretty powerless to contradict them. That's hard, too.*

-Sasha L. AAHCC, CD (eight years)

Now I am so tired of it all, especially the political aspects of hospital birth that I am not taking clients. I really kind of wish I had poured my heart and soul into another career that may have gotten me further ahead financially over the last eight years.

Actually my life feels wrong. I am done doulaing (oh I am so, so done), but am not sure what to fill the space with.

-Michelle, Doula of eight years

Very little discussion of stress and burnout exists in journals and professional literature dedicated to the work of MBPs. Granted, the fields of lactation and labor/postpartum support are in the early stages, as is the resurgence of midwifery. Young professions have a lot of growing pains. As we figure out our place alongside and inside the medical world and with culture at large, there will be stress and conflict. How we understand and face the dangers of stress and burnout will affect the growth and effectiveness of the field. Keeping those with years of experience involved in the mother-baby field provides a historical context and level of wisdom that isn't there when the majority of professionals are newbies.

What is available suggests that there is a legitimate concern about the stress involved with this type of work. In *Counseling the Nursing Mother: A Lactation Consultant's Guide*, the chapter Professional Considerations, addresses professional burnout, including signs of burnout and suggestions for overcoming burnout (Lauwers & Swisher, 2011). According to Lauwers and Swisher, you must first recognize that the problem of emotional burnout is with the job and not with you. The authors point out that job demands and lack of resources lead to constant psychological overtaxing, exhaustion, and cynicism. As DJ, the lactation consultant quoted earlier said, most of her stress came from her employer, which is often the case with lactation consultants. Many of which are expected to see a large volume of mother-baby pairs and get them successfully breastfeeding, yet they may not have policies or supplies in place to support the breastfeeding challenges their patients face. They may also feel pressure to measure their words carefully in order not to anger others in the working environment or in order to keep getting referrals from a specific care provider. Private practice lactation consultants also struggle with a lack of resources (financial and time) and the added burden of establishing rapport with local pediatricians, obstetricians, and midwives, who may not understand the IBCLC credential. Lactation consultants sometimes feel they must give mothers "constant access," and there seems to be too much work and too little time (Lauwers & Swisher, 2011). They often feel the pressure to be there when mothers call, no matter the time or situation.

Heinig (2009) cautions against a type of self-sabotage leading to burnout that she terms the "do it all" mindset. Hospital lactation departments are notoriously understaffed, and mothers are often seen by other hospital staff (nurses, aides) that may not be as supportive of breastfeeding or trained in breastfeeding management. It can be easy to fall into the trap of wanting to take care of as many mothers as possible or believe that no one can give patients the level of care you give. Just as it seems faster and more effective to pick up your four-year-old's toys instead of teaching him how to do it, it can seem easier to see every mom yourself. However, giving other staff tools and confidence to help breastfeeding mothers, so you don't have to "do it all" and mothers and babies can still be helped in your absence, will empower other staff members and take some of the load off your shoulders. Feeling as if the breastfeeding success of every mother-baby unit depends on you will lead to a crushing level of burden.

Other mother-baby professionals can also feel this type of "do it all" mindset stress. The relatively young doula profession and recent resurgence of midwifery means a shortage of these maternity team members in society. Doulas or midwives may find themselves as the only one in their community or one of a very small group. Mother-baby professionals who know they are the only provider of their type in the community may feel like they can never say no. They may push their calendar to the limit, accepting more clients than they feel like they can handle or scheduling many appointments back-to-back, or even traveling very far from home or office to see mothers because they do not want women or babies to go without the services they offer. Pushing to a state of overload makes it difficult to serve anyone well. Often some help can be given by phone or email, mothers can wait a few days to see us if given a "triage plan," and often there are some resources in the community that can be uncovered. We will discuss strategies to avoid overload in a later chapter.

The Politics of Women's Bodies and Women's Wisdom

Western culture has a clearly defined hierarchy of medical knowledge and wisdom. As birth moved into the hospital, mothering became scientific and woman's wisdom became untrustworthy. The male surgical doctor claimed his role at the top of the pyramid of authority. If you are a total nerd like me, you can find a detailed history of birth and the surrounding controversies by reading *Laboring On* (Simonds, Katz-Rothman, & Norman, 2006) and *Birth as an American Rite of Passage* (Davis-Floyd, 1992). Many of us have family stories about someone born at home. My father was the last child in our family to be born at home by the family midwife, his own grandmother. (Two of my children were born at home before I had knowledge that my father had been born at home, too.) Since the 1920's, at least in America, this has been a vanishing family story. Birth and parenthood have been removed from the home, and woman-to-woman passing-of-the-knowledge gave way to things being learned from books and (often male) parenting experts.

Western women having babies today, though perhaps the most educated women in history, are the least experienced or knowledgeable about birth and newborn babies. I was in college before I saw a woman breastfeed, and I was actually a little taken aback that she would do THAT in public! It wasn't until I became pregnant with my first child years later that I learned about breastfeeding for myself. Women are so terrified of birth, the terror has a name–Tokophobia is now being recognized as a distressing psychological disorder. Being socialized to fear the dangers of pregnancy and birth, women are searching for information, but are confused. Combine lack of personal exposure to birth, babies, and breastfeeding with fear and a cultural trust in medicine, surgery, and technology as best, and it makes sense that those of us trying to teach women to follow their bodies and their babies have trouble getting our message across.

That's not to say there isn't research behind lactation consultant strategies, doula care, and midwifery protocols. A quick search of the medical literature will show that research has confirmed much of the wisdom that was passed woman-to-woman for years, and that continues to be passed in many groups around the world. There are complications, however. Lactation consultation is a very young field, first defined in the 1980s, and still working through education requirements, certification requirements, and the controversy of licensure. Doulas work also grew into "paid work" in the 1980s and has had growing pains with the development of several certifying bodies, disagreement over the scope and content of the work itself, and a changing maternity care landscape. Midwives are perhaps the oldest recorded profession; however, they were nearly extinguished in America with the rise of the obstetrician. Midwives have had to rebuild their profession and, at the same time, redefine themselves. These and other mother-baby related professions have been birthed (or re-birthed) to fill the needs of women for support and wisdom. And because these fields are so young, there is still much to be quantified and proven. The new kid on the block, compared to the medical profession that established itself as the leader in the last couple hundred years, has something to prove.

Along with newbie, underdog status, there is the focus on the female mind and body (and that of the child). Within a male dominated society, the value of that which relates to the feminine is lower and sometimes non-existent. All the advances women have made in terms of rights, work, and sexual freedom are difficult to reconcile with the healthcare disparities women face. Women of minority status suffer from even greater healthcare disparities. And even when a woman's physical needs are being tended to by the system, her emotional, mental, and/or spiritual needs may go unmet. Mother-baby professionals hear and sometimes witness mother's stories of mistreatment, disappointment, even trauma. We often work to change hospital policy, educate other professionals and the general public, and increase awareness of the issues. Not arguing or advocating from a place of power, the fight can often seem uphill. Advocacy and activism is often small scale, unfunded, and localized. It can seem as if you are a small voice screaming into a crowd of big voices with megaphones. And with an increasing cesarean rate (up now to 32.9% in 2010) and continued disparities in breastfeeding rates, it can feel as if no one can hear you, no matter how loud you scream.

Mother-baby professionals may also struggle, both internally and externally, with how much to participate in activism. Many who become outspoken are considered "radical." The desire to support women no matter their choices is balanced against what we believe is "best practices." The struggle to support women making different choices than we did or think we would make can be quite difficult for some mother-baby professionals to reconcile. That inner turmoil leads some to restrict their practice to a certain type of client (perhaps who share the same ideals). This is a strategy doulas often employ. We also know that because we may be guests of the family inside the medical system (doulas) or easily fired and replaced (lactation consultants and midwives), we can be removed or threatened if we speak out too often or too loudly. Doulas often talk about playing the "dumb doula" and asking questions of the care provider to get more information for a client instead of giving information or options that might seem to conflict with what the provider is suggesting. Doulas sell their services as advocacy and highlight their training and knowledge, yet some are willing to pretend to be a client's sister if banned from the birth room. Even credentialed homebirth midwives (both nurse and non-nurse) know that prosecution and persecution can be right around the corner if identified on the wrong doctor or health official's radar. Then within certifying and membership organizations, there is much debate over the role of activism, political and financial partnerships, and even licensing/regulation. This can lead to factions and isolationism among practicing professionals, splitting of groups, and further dispersion of power and money. If our key messages and beliefs are scattered individually and personally, it is difficult to move forward toward goals, whatever they might be.

Feeling helpless, isolated, and disconnected, while feeling a high sense of responsibility are signs of chronic stress (Heinig, 2002). Just the nature of being a mother-baby professional can bring about these feelings. It seems built into the very work itself. Won't we always be the underdogs? Won't we always be the new kids on the block? Won't we always feel a high sense of responsibility to the families we serve? Yes, there will always be things we cannot control, but there are ways to deal with these factors that can give power and strength to bring in more positivity and keep stress levels down.

The Current Pace of Life Is Enough to Make You Feel the Burn

The pace of life in Western culture has been on an unstoppable fast track since the industrial revolution. Machines could do our work, the world could become automated, and we would all get more work done in less time! More time for leisure, one would assume. It was a plausible theory indeed. Instead, we now work more and more hours. Our technology has allowed us to be more and more connected. Why wait to return client emails when you can do it at dinner? The price of progress has been the loss of what Dr. Richard A. Swenson calls margin. He explains, "Margin is the space that once existed between ourselves and our limits." Overloaded, too-busy-to-focus lives, lives with a lack of margin, is the "nearly universal malady" that we barely notice, let alone know how to cure (Swenson, 2004).

There is an underlying cultural expectation that to be a productive member of society, you are plugged in and doing something at all times. Even if you aren't overloaded and overscheduled, you might feel guilty that you are not. The once sacred (to those keeping religious customs and not) time of weekly rest has disappeared from society. Every extra minute *should* be filled with some type of enriching activity. Many families fill the weekends with classes, activities, sports, meetings, extra work, or other responsibilities. Women, especially mothers, feel a pressure unique to women of our time. Not only do women bring home the bacon and fry it up in the pan (thanks 1970s advertising execs for setting that expectation), we compete to see who can do it with local bacon in a handcrafted pan, served to the kids with kale, while reciting a Spanish poem about pigs! Mommy wars and competitive parenting have led us to this subconscious competition infused into every part of our lives, starting with super-productive busy lives. Kathleen Kendall-Tackett (2005) describes this peer pressure to appear busy all the time in her book, *The Hidden Feelings of Motherhood.* Mothers who are not "constantly on the run" may feel as if they are wasting their time, intelligence, or college education on their little ones. Or perhaps they just feel like they need a more "valid" answer to the question of, "What did you do all day, dear?"

However, tending to a child, fixing meals, taking care of household and adult responsibilities, not to mention the occasional craft or educational activity take up plenty of time in a day. Additionally, you may already have a job outside of the home when your passion is awakened to serve mothers and babies by providing birth and/or breastfeeding related services. And in a field where training may take months or years and many clients find you by word-of-mouth, there is often a time period of working a job or primary career while building your mother-baby business. Those who are able to be at home "full-time" are often juggling multiple activities, such as childcare, a return to college or postgraduate studies, or homeschooling children.

In all our striving and doing in margin-less living, what are we really getting done? Are we pacing our lives or are we just adding more and more to the pile until we are buried under our own responsibilities, interests, activities, and work?

Tips for prospective mother-baby professionals:

- Examine your current amount of "margin." Does life already seem to be at a frantic pace? Find ways to make room for rest, contemplation, and relaxation now as a part of daily life. This may help you form a more accurate picture of how much time you can dedicate to mother-baby work.

- Think about your "ideal" professional and private life. How much time would you like to (or do you have due to responsibilities) spend on home and family? How much time would you like to spend working with young families? Will you spend time driving around or traveling? Will you be satisfied with the number of mothers you can help or be stressed because you cannot serve more each day?

Tips for current mother-baby professionals:

- Think about your life before your mother-baby career. Was it already stuffed to the brim? You may need to look at all areas of your life, not just your work to see where you need to build in margin.

- Accept that there are only 24 hours in each day. How is your time currently divided? Are you satisfied with the amount of time spent serving families and the amount of time spent on family and personal time? If not, how can you redistribute the time to enjoy life more?

The Reality of Work as a Mother-Baby Professional

The sweet smell of a new baby's head, the happy tears and delighted squeals of a new mother, helping a baby latch on for the first time, watching a mother confidently comfort and nurse her baby–these are the "highs," the rushes of oxytocin, the moments when you know you have been a part of someone else's miracle.

But as is often the case with helping professions, the hours are long and the emotional demands can be high. With the unpredictable life of someone who receives all or part of their work while "on call"–never knowing who or what will be on the other end of the phone–managing personal and professional responsibilities can be a challenge. Add that to the fact that your friends and family always ride the mother-baby professional roller coaster, too–never knowing if you will be attending a birthday dinner or called away from your girls' night out can strain even the most solid relationships.

Kate, a lactation consultant, sums it up well:

> *Giving so much, so often, of yourself with your clients/ patients makes you feel you have less to give to yourself and/ or family. In this line of work, we are all caregivers, social workers, counselors, and ministers even. You are caring for not just mom & baby, but the whole family. That is exhausting!*
>
> - Kate Cropp, RNC, IBCLC, MSN, HCHI

Characteristics of life as a mother-baby professional:[2]

- Being on-call (availability may vary, but for many this means being available by phone, email, or text at all times).

- Interrupted activities – any activity you are engaged in may be interrupted by a phone call, which may, in turn, mean you have to go. Unless you block out entire days, weeks, or months, you may miss family events, such as birthdays, parties, and anniversaries.

- Explaining yourself–Doulas often have to tell people how to pronounce the word, let alone explain the concept. Lactation consultants may get asked, "How hard can it be to breastfeed? We need specialists for that?"

---

2   There are many factors and variations depending on individual situations. This is just a general overview based on my experience and conversations with doulas, childbirth educators, midwives, and lactation consultants.

Midwives may get asked if they have any training at all or why a woman wouldn't just go to a doctor who can "do it all."

- Preparedness – being prepared to go to work as needed instead of always clocking in and out at a specific time. Supplies may not always (or often) be provided for you, and you need to purchase and keep your supplies prepared at all times.

- May have to communicate with caregivers or staff members who may not understand or appreciate the services you provide.

- Expenses, such as continuing education, supplies for clients and self while working.

- Dedication to a profession dealing with women and children – cultural groups with little social status, power, and often low financial resources. It can be difficult to advocate for them in the healthcare system. This in itself is a unique stressor.

- Constant learning and growth. This is a good thing! Your mind is constantly growing and expanding; this is not a career path that includes many "mindless tasks." Be prepared to stretch your brain each day!

- Uncertainty due to the "auxiliary" nature of the work. Labor support and lactation support are rarely provided by hospitals and are not regarded as moneymakers when provided. They are often the first to go when a budget item needs to be cut. Even well liked midwifery programs are sometimes the victim of budget cuts or other hospital politics. And self-employed mother-baby professionals know that families may not choose our services unless they can get insurance reimbursement, even if it will save them money in the long run.

- Emotionally charged work – mothers come to us during vulnerable, emotional times – pregnancy, labor, and postpartum. The empathy we show is crucial to helping mothers feel understood and helped; however, it requires us to be in touch with and in control of the emotions going on inside ourselves.

- Low pay for a healthcare related profession. Most people do this work for many reasons – financial reward NOT being one of them. While you can make a living serving mothers and babies, it may take a long time to build a client base, and it takes discipline and business skill.

Chapter 2

"In most cases, stress is the root cause of death; illnesses are just the wrap up."

-Yordan Yordanov

Levels of Heat: Understanding the Six Flames That Can Destroy Your Passion

Everyone will experience stress in life. As far as level of heat, daily stress is a small flame, like the flicker of a candle. Whether we work in the mother-baby world or not, just being a person exposes us to stress, and we produce a stress response. Stress is good for us. Yes, I just said, stress is good for us human beings. It's that little light from a candle that we need. Speaking in front of a crowd, confronting someone about a concern, playing a timed game on a computer, skiing down a slope, or even playing sports–all of these activities can cause stress. Our stress response, driven by hormones, consists of more rapid heart rate and breathing, tightened muscles ready to activate, sharper senses, and more, as your body's neurological system kicks into gear. This is great if you need to be quick on your feet, make quick decisions, or face your fears. In real or imagined threats or stressful situations, the stress produces a response from our bodies that helps us meet the challenge. However, that response is designed to be short lived. The stress comes, we respond and meet the challenge, and then return to a state of regular body function and activity, such as sleeping, eating, and interacting with others. All of those regular activities are challenged when the stress response is turned on. So while stress is normal and part of our body's natural function, it can also hurt if experienced at high levels and chronically over the course of time.

As we open up this discussion, it is important that we have a basic understanding of the levels and types of stress helpers encounter. The following definitions lay the foundation for grasping the problem as it relates to mother-baby professionals.

The First Flame: Stress

Stress is any threat, danger, or discomfort, real or imagined, mental or physical that activates the stress response in your body.

The stress response activates your nervous system to release "stress" hormones, such as adrenaline and cortisol, which prepare the body for immediate action. This is also referred to as the "fight or flight" syndrome (men) or "tend and befriend" syndrome (women).

The stress response is immediate, rapid, and automatic. Your stress response is highly effective, but it works just as well for a physical threat, like dodging a punch to the face, and an emotional threat, such as receiving several large unexpected bills in the mail. Having many mental stresses can bring on the stress response and keep it there for long periods. Life in the modern, industrialized world rarely means stress from an animal attack. Instead it means psychological stress from a wide variety of internal and external pressures. Parenting in isolation, economic strain, and unhealthy relationships–the list goes on and continues throughout life. This chronic stress, living with prolonged emotional and mental stress, can expose the body to long-term stress response hormones, such as adrenaline and cortisol. Health problems, such as higher blood pressure, higher risk of heart attack and stroke, compromised immune system, decreased fertility, and more, can result from the way chronic stress disrupts most of the body's systems (Smith, Jaffe-Gill, & Segal 2010). Depression, anxiety, and sleep problems–conditions that often occur together–are also common consequences of continued stress response (Smith et al., 2010).

Whether you categorize it into the various designations in psychological literature or just look at it as plain old stress isn't as important as identifying it and taking steps to mediate the effects.

The most common health problems caused or worsened by stress are (Sapolsky, 2011):

- Cardiovascular disease and hypertension

- Depression and anxiety

- Sexual dysfunction

- Infertility, irregular menstrual cycles

- Erectile dysfunction

- Frequent colds

- Sleeplessness and fatigue

- Trouble concentrating

- Memory loss

- Appetite changes

Your body is the physical component of who you are, the instrument with which you do your work. And much of mother-baby work is hands-on. We need our bodies to cooperate with us to do what we do. That said, our bodies are often what we neglect the most and feel worst about. Sleep is optional, aches and pains are ignored, and physical activity is a luxury. When I look around at conferences, I see a bunch of exhausted and overweight people, coming to learn how they can help others more! Ouch. Harsh? Maybe, but trust me, I am right there with you, and I know the deep consequences of taking care of yourself last. Your body WILL wake you up one day. Don't wait until you are on week ten of a sinus infection to realize that you are suffering from an immune system impaired by stress.

The consequences of stress on your physical body can be long lasting, and sometimes permanent. There is a growing body of research to support the idea that your physical body, longevity, and incidence of disease are all impacted by stress. Chronic stress is most damaging and is shifting the focus on healthy living to a more well-rounded approach. Our bodies need proper nutrition and exercise for physical activity, but our bodies need us to pay attention to stress levels, too. For years, many holistic care providers have warned that chronic stress can lead to hormonal imbalance, such as thyroid dysfunction and adrenal fatigue. Just now gaining steam in mainstream medicine, a growing number of people are finding answers when a combination approach of addressing hormones, diet, physical activity, and mental health is used.

As we discuss different types of stress, it is important to know that while specific constellations of symptoms might constitute a specific diagnosis or treatment plan, you don't have to have a technical psychological diagnosis in order to begin facing your stress and attempting to lessen it. However, if you feel as though you would benefit from professional help, please seek the counsel of a trained and licensed counselor, psychologist, or therapist. Your emotional and mental health is a gift to your family and your clients, and the key to many years of life and meaningful work for you.

Here's a burning tip: Identify what's stressful for you. What may make you a nervous wreck may make someone else feel alive and positively challenged! Embrace what works for you and don't worry about if it is different for someone else! Take a day (or a week) and make note of people, situations, or things that produce a stress response in you. Write down how you felt, acted, and even what made you feel better. See what patterns develop and get to know your relationship to stress better. You may find some things you are doing make your stress worse or that you already have some great stress relief strategies.

Only you know what things produce a stress response in your body and how much stress is too much. It is important to understand the role your own thoughts play into your stress level. We will discuss self-care strategies for dealing with daily stresses in part three of this book. Next we move on to Secondary Stress (also called secondary trauma or vicarious trauma).

Secondary stress and/or trauma have been identified in therapists, helpers, and medical and allied healthcare providers. Mother-baby professionals are easily identified as helpers and can deal with this same type of stress.

The Second Flame: Secondary Stress

Secondary stress can be as simple as "stress caused by pressures placed on professionals who care for others in need" (Wicks, 2006). MBPs, by definition, care for others in need. Women in the perinatal period, although not sick, are in a special place of need. Their bodies are going through numerous hormonal and physical changes, along with the emotional rollercoaster of the early days of motherhood. They can be strong and assertive one moment and vulnerable and unsure the next. A pregnant, birthing, or postpartum woman is in a state of emotional (such as support for her choices or dealing with emotions from her own childhood) and/or physical (someone to lean on during birth or help for damaged nipples) need, and mother-baby professionals help to care for those needs. Then there is the baby. If anyone needs the help of others, it is an entirely helpless baby. MBPs are generally helping the baby as well. This pressure on professionals is a mixture of institutional, personal, and situational. Identifying and appreciating secondary stress is important for developing a personal self-care plan and long-term strategies to deal with the stresses inherent with caring for new parents and babies.

Others refer to **Secondary Traumatic Stress** (STS) as "work related, secondary exposure to extremely stressful events" (proqol.org, 2011). The key element of secondary traumatic stress (also called secondary traumatization) is fear (Larsen, Stamm, & Davis, 2002). Symptoms, such as fearfulness, flashes of upsetting images, trouble sleeping, or avoiding anything that might remind one of the event, can come on suddenly and are typically associated with a particular event.

Let me take a short detour and explain a little about the word trauma. I do not want to lightly extract information from psychological literature focused on helpers who help with disaster relief and crises, and apply them to our work as mother-baby professionals. Trauma comes from the Greek word for wound. The modern word has stayed true to its lineage – now understood to mean emotional or physical shock, injury, or pain that may have long-lasting effects. Just working with moms and babies will not land you in the path of trauma or STS; however, there is the possibility of encountering it in the course of your career. Those supporting women during labor and delivery are at highest risk due to the life and death circumstances surrounding birth today.

Birth Trauma

Recently terms such as *birth trauma, postpartum posttraumatic stress disorder (PPTSD)*, and even *birth rape* have come into the maternal health discourse. Birth trauma commonly means either postpartum PTSD, as it is defined by the clinical criteria, or some of the symptoms of PTSD suffered by a woman due to experiences before, during, or directly after childbirth. But isn't birth a wonderful event that ends with a beautiful baby and the wonderful experience of parenthood? For some, maybe most – yes. Motherhood has its challenges, but it is filled with joy. However, for some women, birth becomes a nightmare that meets the definition of a traumatic event.

Many women feel as though they are experiencing some of the nine symptoms required for a clinical diagnosis of PTSD after birth. They may not fit the full definition, yet they are still struggling with disturbing traumatic stress. It is possible you might notice clients who have some of these symptoms or suffer from them yourself. If you suspect a client has any of these symptoms in relation to her birth experience, it is important to refer them to an appropriate licensed mental healthcare provider.

According to **TABS** (Trauma and Birth Stress, a *Charitable Trust based in New Zealand; 2011)*, these symptoms should alert you to possible PTSD:

- Experienced an event perceived by the person experiencing it as traumatic

- Flashbacks of the event, vivid and sudden memories

- Nightmares of the event

- Inability to recall an important aspect of the event - psychogenic amnesia

- Exaggerated startle response, constantly living on edge

- Hyper-arousal, always on guard

- Hyper-vigilant, constantly looking around for trouble or stressors

- Avoidance of all reminders of the traumatic event

- Intense psychological stress at exposure to events that resemble the traumatic event

- Physiological reactivity on exposure to events resembling the traumatic event - panic attacks, sweating, palpitations

- Fantasies of retaliation

- Cynicism and distrust of authority figures and public institutions

- Hypersensitivity to injustice

Even with the high rate of interventions and surgical birth today, most women are not having these symptoms after vaginal or cesarean deliveries. However, a percentage of women *are* feeling traumatized by their birth experiences and postpartum experiences. These women are beginning to find each other and form groups for awareness and support. They are letting the world know birth was anything but a joyful event for them. Women, whether fitting the definition of PTSD or recognizing some sort of postpartum mood disturbance, are starting to recognize something wasn't right. Mother-baby professionals supporting them may very well come to realize that they don't feel quite right either, perhaps dealing with a trauma or extreme stress of their own.

Solace for Mothers, an organization dedicated to healing after traumatic childbirth, explains it by saying:

> *When a woman looks forward to giving birth to a baby, she may not know exactly how the birth will go, but she has a basic expectation of respectful and protective treatment from her partner and from maternity care providers. This expectation includes the right to understand and to participate in health care decisions, and a confidence in her and baby's safety. When these things are not present, the results can be severe.*

- www.solaceformothers.com

Solace for Mothers and other organizations, such as the Birth Trauma Association, the Birth Crisis Network, Birth Trauma Canada, and TABS, acknowledge that birth trauma impacts witnesses to the birth, as well. Some groups offer support for birth partners and fathers, but support for those who professionally attend birthing women does not seem to be offered by any of these organizations. Sheila Kitzinger, well-known British childbirth advocate, social anthropologist, and founder of Birth Crisis teaches workshops where mother-baby professionals can learn to counsel women who have experienced birth trauma. But what about the MBP who feels traumatized?

While most MBPs have a personal belief in natural, low intervention birth, and immediate and long-term breastfeeding as the ideal for healthy women, the reality of birth in Western culture, especially in the United States, is much different. With an overall cesarean rate of 32.9% that has risen for the 13th consecutive year and the fact that artificial rupture of membranes is the ninth most common hospital procedure, we can guess that MBPs are often attending births that go against the ideals they hold. For most mother-baby professionals, most of the time, these normal but not natural births can be balanced by the "good births," the births where mothers feel empowered and a part of the decision-making process, no matter how they gave birth or what interventions were performed. Even if emotionally draining, the MBP can recover with a few days of rest, rejuvenating activities, and a talk with a friend or spouse. It is the births that include something more disturbing, be it harsh treatment of the mother by the hospital staff, forced procedures, an uncontrolled postpartum hemorrhage, maternal death, fetal or newborn death, or other emotional or physical event that can turn a simple stressful element of mother support into a very traumatic event for the doula or midwife.

While stress is not always at the level of trauma, there are many mother-baby professionals who would describe much of what mothers are going through during birth and the early days of motherhood as traumatic. The incidence of traumatic birth may be as high as 34%, with some women experiencing symptoms of PTSD (Simkin, 2004). Women tell stories of forced cesareans, use the term "birth rape," and talk about their traumatic experiences online and at support group meetings, such as ICAN (International Cesarean Awareness Network) or Trust Birth. If mothers are experiencing trauma, it is no surprise that those who intimately support them might be experiencing trauma, as well.

Tracy and Teresa, both experienced doulas, were impacted by the trauma of baby loss:

> *Having lost a baby during labor with a client- it was stressful to even trust birth for several births later...after the birth, I called a mentor who told me to take time to care for myself. For the next five to six births, I was much more comfortable when we were keeping track of mom and baby's heartbeat during pushing (when the other baby had been lost).*

Teresa Howard, CLD, CLE, CCCE, CHBE

After the stillbirth of my third child, I, perhaps foolishly, continued to take clients until I found I was pregnant again five months later. At this point, I knew I needed some time off, but expected to take clients again when this new baby was about six months old. However, after [attending] a 36 hour labor (while I was still exclusively breastfeeding!), I realized that my family needed me more than anyone else's family. So, for about three years, I focused on my Lamaze classes and only took a few "special" clients, like VBAC moms or my students. This enabled me to care for my growing family and bring some balance, healing, and sanity back into my life.

Tracy Good, CD(DONA), LCCE

I also know what it's like to wake up the morning after seeing a lifeless baby in the arms of his mother. It's the type of moment that makes you question everything you have ever believed about women's bodies and the wisdom of birth. I had never been to a conference session about "adverse outcomes" or heard a doula trainer discuss fetal demise, but here I was, shocked by the grief and heartache over losing a baby that wasn't even mine to lose. It can be the event that does a doula's or midwife's passion in. We all know it can happen, but can't bear to let our minds go there. It (along with a long list of other stressors) led to my breaking point, in part, because I was already so weak from overwork and a lack of self-care. Having a self-care plan in place and a way to grieve with friends, mentors, and family may make the difference in the impact of this type of event for the mother-baby professional.

So while not every doula or midwife will witness a traumatic birth event in his or her career, it is important to discuss. Lactation consultants may also face this if they are seeing mothers bedside in a hospital or in early postpartum; however, not being involved in the life and death of the birth process, the exposure would be more limited.

If you have unresolved stress symptoms that meet some of the criteria for PTSD, it is possible that you could be suffering from some type of secondary or vicarious traumatization, especially if you can trace it to a specific event or series of events when supporting mothers during birth. Making this discovery requires careful examination, identification, counseling, and therapy. Helpful therapy may include EMDR (Eye Movement Desensitization and Reprocessing) and hypnotherapy. With many MBPs in competitive environments or isolated, it is important to find or build a network, mentor, find online communities, or contact mothers' groups, such as Solace for Mothers, for information and support.

Again, it is important to understand what might be considered a traumatic event, so you can recognize when you may be affected by it. It is important to differentiate between stressful situations, burnout from lack of support, working too hard, etc., and a traumatic event that changes your entire outlook on life and the work you do. Knowing the difference will go a long way in helping you develop and execute your personal care plan for emotional health.

Rothschild (2006) describes two types of secondary traumatization. The first type of secondary trauma occurs due to the close relationship with the one who has experienced the trauma (even if the non-victim wasn't there). While the trauma is not occurring to the person himself or herself, their close relationship with the victim makes it "hurt" them, too. This aligns with the previously given definitions and is probably the most common understanding of secondary trauma. Doulas and midwives are probably more likely to deal with this type of secondary trauma, as they may form a family-like relationship with their clients during pregnancy.

The second type of secondary trauma is eyewitness trauma. Again, the trauma is happening to someone else–the mother, baby, or father/partner in this case, but the mother-baby professional is there to witness it. This is different from vicarious trauma, which we will discuss next because it is a "direct experience." It may include primary trauma, as well as something that may be happening to the professional while they are witnessing the trauma to the primary victim(s).

An example of this might be a doula supporting a mother during a birth in which the baby is lost during the labor. It is the mother and father (or other partner/family members there) whose baby has died. It is that mother's horror and ultimate nightmare, but it is a terrible tragedy to watch as a lifeless baby is placed into a mother's arms. The doula is typically the person in the room who has spent the most time with this family in long prenatal visits and knows their deepest wishes and desires for their birth. She is an eyewitness to the trauma of losing a baby and may also be traumatized herself at witnessing the tragic death of a baby during birth. This could qualify under the standard or first type of secondary trauma, as well as just giving care to someone in this stressful, traumatic situation would also impact the doula.

The Third Flame: Vicarious Trauma

Vicarious trauma is "second-hand" trauma from hearing about the stressful and/or traumatic experience of someone else, and imagining or feeling their pain. Even though you were not present during the event, you can still vicariously experience it in your own nervous system when you hear the story (Rothschild, 2006). Think about the phrase, "I feel your pain." You don't *really* feel the pain of another person. You are empathizing, taking on how they feel. A mother-baby professional might "feel the pain" of a client telling them about an experience or mistreatment.

A lactation consultant might suffer from vicarious trauma after a consultation with a mother who had a very negative birth experience, leading to complications that affected the ability to breastfeed, and was followed by poor breastfeeding advice. I once had a client whose three-week-old exclusively breastfed baby had not gained weight in one week. He was brought back in from being weighed at the pediatrician's office with a bottle of formula in his mouth – without her prior consent. Now, whether this mother may have needed to supplement the baby is irrelevant. They did not consult the mother before feeding her baby formula for the first time. Perhaps she had pumped milk with her, could feed her baby right away, or had a preference as to what she wanted to feed her baby – the point is they took action before a brief consultation with the perfectly competent mother. I was so angry for this mother! So angry I wanted to scream! It didn't happen to my baby or me, but I had an immediate, strong stress response and wanted to "fight" for that mom and baby. Many lactation consultants seeing mothers who have been the recipients of incorrect lactation advice experience this type of "second hand" stress (fueled by outrage) regularly, especially when they are in a particularly nonbreastfeeding-friendly environment.

The Fourth Flame: Compassion Fatigue

Compassion Fatigue is "the negative aspect of our work as helpers" (Proqol, 2011). According to the developers of the ProQOL (2011) measure, burnout and secondary trauma are elements of compassion fatigue. MBPs suffering from compassion fatigue may have either or both burnout and secondary trauma of some sort. Compassion fatigue is also described as chronic secondary stress and suffering from helping work, and is sometimes used interchangeably with burnout (Wicks, 2006). Descriptions vary in the mental health community of compassion fatigue and its relationship to burnout. Both compassion fatigue and burnout are primarily defined by the chronic, continued feeling of stress and pressure.

The Fifth Flame: Burnout

Burnout has many descriptions in mental health literature. Wicks (2006) describes burnout as "chronic secondary stress." Rothschild's definition of burnout is more descriptive. When a person's physical health or life outlook is impacted to the point of negativity overload, that is burnout. Unlike secondary traumatic stress, burnout generally comes on gradually (Proqol, 2011). It's as if you have more and more negative thoughts until you no longer feel as if your work is making a difference. Feelings of hopelessness and an inability to do your work may ensue. Some may struggle with burnout due to very high amounts of work or lack of support in the workplace. While for others, burnout may be triggered by the overwhelming emotional stress of helping others with intense situations.

Burnout is a very real concern for the MBP due to the nature of the work. Birth workers (doulas and midwives) spend many hours in the very physical and emotional work of supporting a laboring woman. While the work may not come every day (though it may for some working in a hospital environment), it is intense and unpredictable when it does come. Lactation-focused MBPs deal with these issues or some variation, as well. Workloads for MBPs are often high due to solo or small group practice, feelings of guilt about turning people away, or being the only provider in the area. Lack of support (or lack of *feeling* support) in the workplace is a reality for those in hospital settings, as they may be the only one or one of a small group of people doing their job. Private practice MBPs may also feel lack of support when they participate in the hospital environment, supporting their clients, or are interacting with other members of the mother's or baby's healthcare team. The cultural lack of support for women and women's work may also be a factor in burnout for those passionate about the uniquely feminine tasks of birth, breastfeeding, and mothering.

The Sixth Flame: Depression

Depression is the consuming fire that destroys all joy from life. Depression can be a symptom or a result of too much stress, of being burned out, or of experiencing trauma (first hand or secondary). Feeling hopeless, sleepless, extreme sleepiness, and loss of joy from regularly enjoyable activities are all clues that depression may have taken hold in your mind. Depression has been described as living in darkness by some or feeling an overall heaviness or emptiness – a heartache that won't let you go. And for some, it can lead to a strong desire to get out by ending the life that is so full of pain. Depression can take your life or severely limit life quality for yourself and those that love you. It is important to recognize it either as a piece of other stress problems or as a problem within itself.

Identify It and Face It

All of these concepts are interwoven. One can lead to another or several types can be present together, creating deep emotional and physical damage. Stress in all the aforementioned varieties affects your quality of life–both professionally and personally. We must take care of ourselves if we truly desire to give the best care to those we serve.

Identifying what type of stress you are experiencing is not as important as facing the fact that you are having it. If you see yourself being burned by any of the six flames of stress discussed here, seek the assistance of a skilled mental healthcare provider. They can help you work through the stress and put into place a self-care plan that will lead to long-term health. Self-help books are great–I'm writing one I guess, but for some, working with a mental health professional will create the greatest, long-lasting results.

Chapter 3

Empathy – The Kindling of Burnout or the Flame of Passionate Work?

"Stress is like an iceberg. We can see one-eighth of it above, but what about what's below."

-Author Unknown

What if keeping the six flames under control is not just about time management, learning to relax, and developing personal care plans? Perhaps we also need to look at our basic humanity, at the gift of passion and care for others. The very fire that makes us passionate about moms and babies can also be a contributing factor in what can lead to states of stress and burnout. Empathy is that very fire inside of us that makes us want to help mothers and babies. We empathize with the new mother who loves her baby so much her heart aches. We feel it and want to support her, cheer her on, and give her good information. But that fire of empathy, when fanned by negative or traumatic events, can lead to stress and burnout in the professional helper. Learning how empathy plays a role in our work with mothers and babies can help us develop strategies to keep the stress of caring for others to a minimum.

How Empathy Affects Your Work

Fire needs something to burn–it doesn't just appear out of the air. Kindling is the material used to start a fire. Empathy is the emotional and mental experience used to create the six flames we have discussed–stress, STS, vicarious trauma, compassion fatigue, burnout, and depression. Empathy is how we feel the pain and distress of another. Empathy is why you get bummed out when your spouse is all bummed out after a rough day at work. Empathy is why you tense your muscles when you watch your child shoot a basketball during a game. Empathy is powerful. Feeling the feelings of another–empathy–can hurt you, but it is also an essential part of what makes us human.

Psychological professionals define empathy in numerous ways. For our purposes here, I will share with you two definitions that speak specifically to our work as helpers.

From the Merriam-Webster's Medical Dictionary at Dictionary.com (2011):

> The action of understanding, being aware of, being sensitive to, and vicariously experiencing the feelings, thoughts, and experience of another of either the past or present without having the feelings, thoughts, and experience fully communicated in an objectively explicit manner.

And from The American Heritage® New Dictionary of Cultural Literacy, Third Edition (2011):

> Identifying oneself completely with an object or person, sometimes even to the point of responding physically, as when, watching a baseball player swing at a pitch, one feels one's own muscles flex.

By definition, empathy isn't all bad, right? It seems to be a double-edged sword. Empathy can kick you into secondary traumatic stress when a client loses a baby, but it is also what allows you to share in the height of joy when a new baby offers her first cry. Rothschild (2006) describes empathy as "necessary for the survival of the species." It is what makes us human, what allows us to respond to the needs and desires of others. Empathy allows you to feel the thrills and joys of another. However, empathy unchecked, unaware, can cause damage to the MBP's mind, soul, and body.

Most of the time empathy is automatic and unconscious. A friend smiles at you and you smile back. You might feel they are having pleasant feelings, then when you mimic their smile–that is a physical (somatic) empathy, you might also have pleasant feelings–that is emotional empathy. Think about it the next time you return the smile of a stranger at the grocery store. You do it automatically, and your mood lifts at least a little. Empathy allows you to feel those positive feelings and change your face to mimic another.

Physical and emotional empathy are closely linked. What sometimes starts as mimicking a client's body posture or facial expression can lead to experiencing feelings similar to what they are feeling, or what you think they are feeling, and vice versa. Physical empathy is when you feel the physical feelings of another. It's why mothers have a difficult time watching their little boy get tackled on the football field. It's the reason you scrunch up your face when you see someone get slapped. This happens with emotions, as well. When you notice someone with a sad look on his or her face, generally you change your countenance, quiet your voice, and speak in a different tone than you would if the person were smiling. This is why mothers might describe their doula, midwife, or lactation consultant as "knowing just what I felt," that feeling of synchronicity that occurs when human beings connect deeply with each other. It is a complicated neurological process with volumes of books dedicated to its understanding. While empathy is a natural process, it affects each of us differently. Those who most closely empathize with their clients are at highest risk of compassion fatigue (Rothschild, 2006). Empathy is an essential part of your work with mothers, but it can also lead to identifying so closely that the physical and emotional sensations and realities they feel become something you feel, too.

In the case of our work with pregnant, birthing, and postpartum women, it is important that we empathize with them. We want to validate their feelings, show them kindness, and create a safe space for them to share their feelings. Being able to recognize how and when you empathize with clients and when it creates too much distress in your body and mind is a powerful way to turn down the heat. We don't want to become robot helpers, with no emotion in our eyes, but it is important that we are able to offer a calm, comforting response without doing damage to ourselves. Is it ever okay to cry with a client? To be angry? Jumping up and down excited? Absolutely. But there are other times when they will need us to hold it together or our professionalism demands it, so we must be able to empathize without losing ourselves to the emotions that belong to our client. It's not just about maintaining a professional distance; taking home the emotions of the client can be like bringing home a storm cloud that sits over the rest of your life.

For example, Lucy Lactation Consultant, an IBCLC, has a consultation with a young mother of a five-day-old baby who doesn't seem to be gaining weight well. The mother is tearful throughout the consultation, terrified that she is starving her baby and desperate to be able to feed her baby at the breast. After the consultation, Lucy goes home and struggles to find the energy to make dinner. When her husband comes home, she feels sad, down, and exhausted. What's wrong with Lucy? Her empathy for the young mother has taken over. She so closely identified with the young mother that she took her feelings home with her.

Most of the time, we are able to shake off unconscious empathy, and we don't keep the feelings of others on us for long. You might be able to sit down with someone and identify an interaction with a client or co-worker (or someone else) that has changed your mood. But it can build, especially if we are unaware of the source. It can be internalized and seen as negativity, chronic bad mood, or your own feelings. At a doula training I attended in 2010, an attendee described how deeply the hormones and emotions of birth affected her at the very first birth she attended. When she first started experiencing births, the rush of oxytocin was so overwhelming that she couldn't help but rush home and passionately make love to her boyfriend. She had no idea what made her so amorous, and for a while she never connected the two "activities." She also explained that "bad births" sent her for a soak in the tub and a few days of emotional recovery. Now further along in her doula career, she could recognize the strong impact of birth hormones and emotions on herself and handle her feelings and choose actions accordingly.

Being aware of your empathetic response and its effect on your body, mind, and spirit will be helpful in keeping your regular stress levels low. Am I saying NOT to empathize with your clients? Not at all! In fact, it is the essence of what we do. Can you see it now? A doula is face-to-face with a mother. She rocks and moans as the mother rocks and moans. A midwife's tears fall as the mother's eyes overflow as she births her long awaited baby, or the lactation consultant who breathes a deep cleansing breath with a scared woman who last week was a high powered executive, but this week is the mother of a 6 lb 4 oz baby who won't latch. We show empathy to these women and all the women we serve. We keep the fire contained by learning to recognize and harness it for the good of our clients and ourselves.

Dr. Ellie Izzo and Vicki Carpel Miller (2009) of the Vicarious Trauma Institute (Vicarioustrauma.com) hold a differing theory. They propose that it is the controlling of empathy that actually leads to vicarious trauma. The theory holds that the complex neurological process of empathy is short-circuited when we are not able to express the reaction that hearing a traumatic story (such as when a woman tells you an awful, traumatic birth story) produces. They suggest that suppressing those emotions and reactions (perhaps due to a need to remain professional and not react) leads to negative physical, emotional, and spiritual consequences. Suppressing your emotions would not be considered healthy in most cases, so it makes sense that suppressing your empathetic responses might negatively affect your body, mind, and spirit. In that case, learning to create outlets where you can let out those responses (by discussing a case with another trusted professional perhaps) and finding ways to nurture your emotional, physical, and spiritual self is highly important.

Perhaps the answer lies somewhere between the given theories. It is important to be aware of your body posture, muscle tension or relaxation, facial expressions, thoughts, emotions, and energy level when with clients. Do certain clients or types of clients "drain" you? Do you always get a headache or stomachache after meeting with a specific client? Do you notice yourself clenching your hands or jaw or breathing differently as you work with clients? After leaving a client, do you feel anxious, angry, upset, calm, or joyful? What are your feelings based on? How your client felt or pride about the service you provided? Take a moment to think about how you feel after work. Do you remember having particularly strong sensations in your body and/or emotions after working? Perhaps you were empathizing with her so deeply that you were really "feelin' it" as the saying goes. In the next section, we will discuss strategies to harness your empathy for the good of both yourself and your clients.

You should feel positive about your interactions with your clients and the work you do. This is good, meaningful work. Even a job with stressors can leave you with a sense of joy when you are able to manage your emotions and stress response. One of my mentors, Teresa Howard, a former La Leche League leader, childbirth educator, doula, and trainer, with years of experience, has given me many words of wisdom over the years. She said there are times when we need to step away from our work, be it for a few hours, days, or a month or more. When we are caring for women, we have to be careful not to care more (about her having a natural birth or exclusively breastfeeding, for example) than the woman cares about it, meaning we can't want it for her. Whatever is meant to be for that mom is meant to be. Thinking you can will things to happen a certain way because you want it for her will only lead to burnout for you. In 15 years, Teresa has assisted nearly 500 births, helped hundreds more breastfeed, and survived breast cancer. Her advice about overcoming stress has been tested by fire. She is an example of a MBP who has learned to mediate stress and adapt her work and life to avoid burnout.

Compounders - Thinking About Your Past and Your Present

We have discussed stressors—causes of stress from family needs to work responsibilities to conflict with others. What causes a stress response in one person may not even be an irritation to another person. Situations from your past, your current life situation, and even what you may anticipate in your future can also play a part in how you respond to stressors. Many mother-baby professionals are mothers themselves. Your past experiences are a filter for all the education and training you receive.

Our greatest hurts sometimes become our greatest source of strength for helping others. Each person must work through her past in order to pull from it what can help others. Working with women going through the same events (birth and breastfeeding) that you may have struggled with can bring up feelings that compound an already stressful event. Memories of an event you may have "dealt with" long ago can come to the forefront as you see a woman in a similar place.

Helping a woman through a situation you are currently dealing with or think you might deal with can bring up feelings of "what if this happens to me?"

Feelings of vulnerability may creep in as you think about the similarities between you and your client. These are all things to keep in mind as you think about the physical and emotional responses you have to your clients. Are you feeling stress that is compounded by current circumstances or events from your past? Exploring who you are and what has happened in your life is a valuable part of knowing yourself as a professional. It will help you identify and modify stress if you know what may compound the stress caused by situations and people you encounter.

Chapter 4

Why Mother-Baby Professionals?

"Reality is the leading cause of stress for those in touch with it."

-Jane Wagner

There are issues unique to the world of mother-baby professionals that make our work stressful and likely to lead to burnout. This section will address the unique challenges that make life as a mother-baby professional vulnerable to stress. By identifying these challenges we will be able to confront them and make changes when the burn is too hot to handle.

Who we are, what work we do, and where we are in our spheres of influence are all factors in how stress impacts us. Understanding the unique who, what, and where of mother-baby work will help in recognizing and minimizing stress.

Who We Are:	What We Do:	Where We Work – Spheres of Influence:
1. A young, sometimes confused profession	1. Training and education	1. Politics
2. Goddesses with a complex	2. Work with a sense of urgency	2. Power
3. Passionate to the extreme	3. Heart work vs. Bank account work	3. Patient care

Who Do We Think We Are?

 As women (usually) supporting other women in the realm of the uniquely female activities of carrying a child, birthing, and nursing him, the essence of who we are is as old as the human race itself. The wisdom and skills that accompanied such life events were passed down from woman to woman in every village and culture. The professionalization of a woman helping another woman through the perinatal period is fairly new in human history. Even midwives existed more as a revered position of honor and experience versus years of academics, training, and business structure.

Formal organizations that certify those who wish to become mother-baby professionals–doulas, lactation consultants, childbirth educators, and non-nurse midwives are a fairly new invention. As childbirth became more and more medicalized and less humane throughout the 1930s and 1950s, and breastfeeding became nearly non-existent, one-by-one mothers, professionals, and activists started to wake up and realize that something was wrong. They began to organize to advocate for the ideals of natural birth, consumer choice, fathers in the delivery room, and less separation of mother and baby. The oldest of these formal organizations are Lamaze (1960), International Childbirth Education Association (ICEA; 1961), and American Academy of Husband Coached Childbirth (AAHCC, also known as Bradley; 1966), which began to certify childbirth educators. Some of these certified educators also attended their students' births as a support person. Birth activists continued to speak out and form parent support groups, such as La Leche League and Informed Home Birth, throughout the 70s. The 1980s brought us the founding of Midwives Alliance of North America (MANA; 1982) and International Board of Lactation Consultant Examiners (IBLCE; 1985), followed by doula certifying organizations–Doulas of North America International (DONA International; 1992) and Childbirth and Postpartum Professionals Association (CAPPA; 1998), and Midwifery Education Accreditation Council (MEAC) for credentialing non-nurse midwives in 1991.

At the most, we can claim fifty years of history–which in the grand scheme of an occupation is not long at all. And most of that time has been spent developing organizations, setting up certification/education pathways, and learning how to interact with the other players in the perinatal field. Many occupations we would consider "professions" (an occupation having formal qualifications based on formal education; skills acquisition under supervision; examinations, along with formal certifying bodies; autonomy; and some level of status and power) such as medicine, law, and accounting, have been solidified since the early 1900s or before. Mother-baby related occupations have struggled to meet the definition of a profession and have had parts, but not all of the factors. At this point in history, IBCLCs, doulas, childbirth educators, and non-nurse midwives fall into a more semi-professional category.

We continue to struggle with what it means to serve mothers and babies as a group. Are these professions that should be licensed and regulated or are they organic and too central to our humanity to be broken down into skill sets and exam questions? Does regulation of those most wise about birth and breastfeeding contribute to the over-medicalization of a universally human experience? The women who wear the various mother-baby professional titles answer these questions individually and collectively. Which organization(s) do you join, if any? Do you become certified or licensed, or not? Are you a hobbyist or a professional? Does professional status mean organizational membership, liability insurance, and a business license or is this a business that is conducted by handshakes and trust? For many, this type of work is about the calling and the heart, not about advertising and making money. And, of course, there are those that would like for it to be about both (I'm in that camp!). Each community also struggles with how to support each other, while also "competing for business." Most MBPs work through these issues alone or in small informal groups, with small, mostly volunteer-run organizations as the only support and "authority." Unlike other professionals, there are no powerful financially backed lobbyists and membership organizations. We exist in a loosely networked weave of membership and certification organizations that don't always play nicely together.

The good and bad news is that the field of mother-baby support has much room for growth. There is much work to be done and lots of passion and energy that could be a force for change if channeled correctly. More organizations are working together to pool resources and unite membership, as evidenced by the Lamaze and ICEA mega-conference in 2010. Grassroots organizations, such as local birth networks and ICAN meetings, are places for professionals with various affiliations, beliefs, and interests to network. More conferences and events held in person and online make it easier to share ideas. Twitter, blogs, and networking websites spread ideas, videos, and conversations quickly, and allow those who might not have been able to enter the dialog before to become involved. More open and rapid communication may be the key to moving forward collectively and moving toward more common goals.

Passionate does not seem like a big enough word to describe what fuels those who give their lives to the service of mothers and babies. For me, it was the deeply satisfying natural birth and successful breastfeeding relationship with my first child that gave me a desire to help other moms achieve birth and breastfeeding goals. For others, their passion for helping mothers is fueled by a desire to help them avoid what they experienced. There is a third, equally passionate group, not motivated by personal experience, but motivated by a deep respect and awe of the process of pregnancy, birth, and/or breastfeeding. No matter the original passionate spark, this is a work path that is far from lined with gold bars. While making a living is a motivation for anyone who calls what they do a job, most MBPs consider what they do to be more about personal satisfaction and service than about becoming wealthy.

We are deeply passionate about deeply private matters: how one carries, births, and nurtures a child. The decisions one makes in the childbearing years are intensely personal, yet carry societal ramifications. I can tell by puzzled looks I sometimes get during dinner party conversations that it can be difficult to understand why someone would so deeply care about the non-medical aspects of pregnancy, birth, and breastfeeding. Why spend so much time helping women with something so "natural?" Can't they just figure it out on their own? At times, it can be discouraging to be so passionate about something that most times exists far out of the mainstream consciousness.

Often a mother-baby professional's personal passions are different from what her clients choose as important for them. There is a complicated dance in combining being deeply passionate about your personal choices, passionately supporting the rights and desires of clients, and offering passionate public advocacy statements. For some, doing all three things is easy, for others finding a way to be passionate in different ways is quite a challenge. Some find their place by opting not to be involved in politics, public discourse, or debate. They focus their passion on their personal life and work with clients. Others have a single focus to their passion and choose to work with a specific client whose passions line up with their personal passions. We have probably all had a job that we did just for the paycheck. Standing on the corner holding a sign for Joe's Furniture Market isn't usually done out of a place of passion. But those getting out of bed at 2:00 a.m. to go to a laboring mother's side or digging in textbooks for information on a mother's disease treatment and her ability to breastfeed are done out of a deep passion to support women and babies.

With all this passion to fuel our desire to help others, we sometimes think we can do this work alone. Due to the popularity of Ricki Lake and Abby Epstein's documentary, *The Business of Being Born*, more women today know about the services provided by midwives and doulas. There are women seeking out birth tubs and exploring their options due to an increased awareness of the broken maternity care system in America. Breastfeeding, at least early breastfeeding, is reaching heights of popularity in many demographic groups of new mothers. It would seem that all this heightened awareness would bring such a great demand that mother-baby professionals would happily share the load. Unfortunately, many doulas, midwives, lactation consultants, and other mother-baby professionals report fierce competition, or what I call the goddess complex.

In group settings at conferences or online, stories are shared about a MBP who takes it upon herself to determine the local going doula fee, discourages newbies, or talks negatively about others in the area. She's the goddess of birth or breastfeeding that all new mothers need by their side. My personal brush with this goddess complex involved a well-established doula who told a potential client that had interviewed with her and our doula group that our group of four doulas worked together because we all had so many children that we couldn't attend our own client's births (so we had to back each other up in case we couldn't leave our children). (I only have three children, and I manage their care just fine, thank you.) If you wish to share about your own family in interviews, that is your business, but to comment on the family choices of another professional, especially in a manner meant to cast doubt on their ability to perform is in bad taste. This episode was an example of the special way women attack each other. It's a two for one attack, calling into question another woman's professionalism and personal decisions. A group of women getting together to share work (and childcare) is actually a great way to provide services and still tend to family. In fact, it is the way most of the world's women have worked throughout history.

In many areas, including my own, tension between non-nurse IBCLCs and nurse (usually hospital-based) IBCLCs is an uncomfortable reality that makes collaboration difficult. IBCLCs from various pathways should have no problem getting along. It is the diversity of training and experience that strengthens the credential. We draw strength from all of our backgrounds, learning from each to teach mothers more. Building a strong connected community means more business for all from referrals, increased public awareness, and more social connections.

In other areas, there is a lack of competition only because of a lack of those providing service. It is challenging to build a community of MBPs when you are the only one or one of just a few. When the number of MBPs is low in a community, then the goddess complex can manifest differently. Some MBPs complain of getting to the point of overload because they can't say no to women wanting services. It may not be a large number of clients, but a doula taking three clients a month might feel maxed out for her family or personal situation. If you are the only IBCLC or independent childbirth educator in your area, you may not be able to help all of the mothers requesting your services. Not having others to refer to in the local area can lead to a feeling of "letting down" the mothers you can't take on as clients. Lactation professionals or others who know that they are the only one in the area who can see mothers in evening or weekend hours may find it difficult to let voice mail answer when sitting down to dinner, even though they don't want to answer the phone.

We must remember that mothers are resourceful. Women are capable. When we build ourselves up as the only help and savior for their crisis moments or support, we put ourselves in a situation of never being able to take a break or say no. You can't be everything to everyone, everywhere at the same time.

Expecting that of yourself is expecting goddess status. Some mother-baby professionals have the goddess complex out of a desire to dominate what they view as a competitive environment; others have it out of a desire to not let a single mother go without help and support. Neither situation is productive or sustainable long-term.

What Is the Work We Do?

Things that have enormous impact on my stress and burnout level: childcare issues, professional bullying, and interfacing with the medical model of birth.

- Lindsey K, CPM, CD, CLC

The path to becoming a mother-baby specialist is different for each of us. For some, it is a path of formal education, such as nursing school, followed by work in mostly medical settings, such as a clinic or hospital. For others, this work starts on a volunteer path, helping friends, family, and community members, and turns into a paid career after self-education. No matter the path, the bulk of the education focuses on technical information and skill acquisition. Very little, if any, time is spent focusing on how to nurture and grow yourself as you give so much of yourself to others.

For breastfeeding helpers, training consists of gaining experience through working with mothers, and education on lactation challenges and norms. You may start out helping women learn proper latch and positioning, and progress to knowledge of the pharmacology involved when medication is in the breastfeeding mother's system. Having received training and education from a variety of organizations and methods, I can attest to the lack of focus on the one providing care. I understand the dilemma—with so much information to learn, it is difficult to cover everything. Dealing with conflict and stress aren't exactly hot conference topics or part of the core curriculum. Sadly, more people will come to workshops dedicated to "infant oral structure and breastfeeding" than "how to nurture yourself." As professionals, we preach that mothers need to take care of their own needs in order to better care for the baby, yet we often ignore our own needs.

Birth professionals are trained in the many ways to assist a mother during pregnancy, birth, and the postpartum period. Over the years, they become walking encyclopedias of information about the stages of labor, birthing choices, and newborn care. A reoccurring complaint I hear about doula training is that very little time is spent on how to run a business. When I have asked doulas and midwives if they received training or information on self-care or burnout prevention, the answer is usually no or that it was gone over briefly. Birth work is extremely satisfying, but also extremely stressful. The idea of taking care of you, as a professional, should be addressed at the career entry point instead of waiting until someone starts to show signs of being overwhelmed. Birth professionals need to be prepared for the stress that has a great possibility of impacting their work and personal life, especially without a plan.

No matter what type of mother-baby work you do, your skills, training, and experience will help you provide excellent care to mothers. We often have to learn "on the job" how to navigate the political world of working with medical care providers. You may have to do your own reading and education to learn to respectfully and courageously speak and act your convictions. Providing evidence-based, factual information is not always accepted and respected. However, giving care that you can be proud of is your duty to yourself. It is your integrity. And, it is something that only you have control over. Integrity is part of your power. You know you are doing right to the best of your ability. With that knowledge, you can give your all to your work, but also give rest and relaxation to yourself. You need times of rest and relaxation in order to be the best at what you do. In the next section of the book, we will discuss strategies for self-care.

Urgency is another factor in the work we do. Babies wait for no man (or woman for that matter). There are times when mothers and babies need the services we offer, and it is not convenient. The on-call lifestyle, the uncertainty of what a day will hold, and not knowing how long the work will take all weigh on the MBP and her family. The needs that arise are needs that cannot be put on hold. For pregnancy and birth related issues, time can be a matter of life or death, whether cesarean section or vaginal birth. In regards to breastfeeding, sometimes a few days can make a tremendous difference in the outcome. Knowing that the work is so time sensitive can set up unrealistic expectations to be immediately available at all times for all clients or potential clients. Realize that this is a source of stress and tension. It's not a personal flaw in you or your family members that a constant on-call life is difficult. Even fire fighters, police officers, and doctors have days and shifts off. You can't be on call ALL the time, but it seems to be the standard. Consider the toll of living in a constant state of urgency, of heightened alert. That keeps you in a constant state of adrenal push! Urgency keeps those emergency hormones always surging. Those glucocorticoids and other hormones are great for dealing with a present danger (running away from an attacker), but cause all sorts of those problems we discussed earlier when stress lingers on a daily basis. Trained to "be there" for our clients, we sometimes do a poor job of setting boundaries and recognizing true urgency from things that can wait. When you lack boundaries or do not hold clients accountable for what they can control, you may feel used and mistreated (Brown, 2010). Compassion for others and boundaries are not mutually exclusive. In the words of Brené Brown (2010), "If we're going to practice acceptance and compassion, we need boundaries and accountability."

Burning Tip: Discipline yourself to NOT respond immediately to email. Your email system should have the ability to set up a vacation responder or auto responder that can send out an automatic response to all who email you. You can use it during particularly busy seasons or as an everyday business tool. Having an automatic response can help lighten the load by easing any anxiety you may have over clients having to wait for a response, by letting the client or potential client know her email was received, and by giving you more time to respond.

An automatic responder example:

Subject: Thanks for the email!

Message: Due to the nature of my work (long appointments with expectant and new families and attending births of various lengths), it may take 24-48 hours to return your email. Thank you for your patience.

Email is checked and returned twice a day. Feel free to call our main number for a more immediate response.

Micky Jones, BS, CLE, CLD, CD(DONA), HCHI, IBCLC contact information

This is just one way to make communication more efficient and less stressful. Of course, you have to follow through by responding to email ONLY twice a day instead of every time your smartphone dings and by taking phone calls when you are able at reasonable times.

A popular saying in the MBP community is that our heart and hands are our most important tools. We "hold the space" to provide room for the mother and baby to find their rhythm in birth or to work out breastfeeding difficulties. So how do you monetize "holding the space" and is it wrong to do so? There are those that passionately believe it is wrong to charge for these types of services and that all clients should be served regardless of ability to pay. There are others who prefer to work for clients who have the means and are happy to pay a premium for the wisdom and service they provide. MBPs struggle personally and professionally with how to balance the need and/ or desire to make money with the belief that women need and deserve the support we offer. The financial bottom line is often cited as a reason for large client loads and "assembly-line" births in our hospitals. If high volume is the only way to make money with the perinatal population, how do MBPs stand a chance? MBPs have to be savvy in order to maximize their earning potential without compromising their standards. Taking every client who comes your way because you need the money will lead to routine mechanical care for the clients you don't connect with. Perhaps specializing in a special type of care (a hypnosis-based childbirth educator offering doula services to clients using that method, for example) or expanding to include other services for consumers or professionals can help pay the bills.

Where Do We Work? – Our Spheres of Influence

Mother-baby professionals live in a land of limbo. There are many places we visit–politics (actual government politics and work related politics), power in our interactions and patient care, but we are always pulled back to the realities of our clients' needs. We also live in limbo between what we believe to be true and optimum, and what our clients often choose to do or let happen to them. In the past, the struggle was clear. Get fathers into the delivery room! Keep mothers and babies together! Now, the struggle is more subtle, more multi-faceted and includes many nuances. Someone who becomes very politically active, involved in protests or legislation, may be branded as radical and not trusted by medical care providers. Someone who challenges what a physician or nurse says may be branded a troublemaker. All of this challenges the heart and emotions. Should I say what I think? Should I be honest when she asks what I know about the doctor she is seeing? What do I say when I know my client is being misled? There are many situations which cause a MBP to question how she will interact with others. How will she assert power? How will she share her knowledge and expertise?

The DONA doula pilot study illustrates some of these issues. Doulas surveyed gave self-critical answers, saying that the role of doula was problematic. They found themselves in conflict while working within the maternity care system (Grant et al., 2010). They noted that many doulas felt uneasy with a limitation on what they felt like they could say and felt intimidated by the hospital system (Grant et al., 2010). Their conclusion was that the challenges doulas face in role and scope need to be addressed, so doulas can gain full acceptance in conventional (i.e., hospital) birth settings (Grant et al., 2010). If doulas address the challenges of their "role and scope," will they gain acceptance? And does gaining acceptance mean that doulas will be able to do their job without conflict and intimidation? What about those already working well within the DONA scope and defined doula role? Most doulas are doing everything they can to walk the line of mother's advocate and nonthreatening member of the birth team. Yet, some providers and hospitals are banning their presence all together. Perhaps the role and scope has changed since the formation of DONA in 1992. The knowledge base and tools available to doulas has certainly changed. This is definitely an issue that needs more exploration and discussion for all mother-baby professionals.

Power in our interactions and patient/client care can also vary based on setting and situation. Many MBPs speak more freely in private patient meetings than in front of medical care providers. MBPs may change what they say or do if they feel there will be negative feedback from care providers. If the caregiver changes your ability to speak to and serve a client, then that changes your care for them. Of course, there is something to be said for adapting to your environment and the other maternity care team members. There is also something to be said for being consistent in what you say and do. Feeling like you constantly have to say the right things in front of the right people without making anyone angry is an impossible situation. You should be able to do what you do with integrity and commitment. If you feel like you can't be a MBP with integrity and commitment, then you should probably make some changes.

There is hope! You can live a life that is full of integrity. You can live a life that has boundaries, is healthy, whole, and low stress. And, you can continue to serve mothers and babies. At first, change is difficult and scary. Even if what you are doing is not working and you are stressed to the max, it might be really frightening to think about making changes. Making changes that honor you, your family, and your clients will give you more joy and less stress. You will be proud of the life you have made for yourself. You may even reap more financial success by being more focused and positive. Taking any of the steps in the next section will help you in the journey to a more peaceful, rewarding, and balanced life if you want a life that honors you as much as it honors the work you do.

Chapter 5

The Six Burn Busters – Controlling the Fire

"Releasing the pressure, it's good for the teapot and the water. Try it sometime."

-Jeb Dickerson

We can all agree that it's important to "take care of yourself" and "recharge your batteries." Unfortunately, no one seems to know what that means, and if they do, they never take time to do it. Avoiding burnout and putting an end to chronic stress entails more than booking the occasional massage or pedicure. The good news is: there are strategies that really work and can help you take control of the stress in your life from everyday living in our fast paced society and from your work as a mother-baby professional.

There are many theories about how to reduce stress and the possibility of burnout in relationship to work. Sometimes just thinking about the things you should be doing to relieve stress are enough to stress you out. When I was at the height of my darkest, stress-induced time, putting "personal time" on my ever-growing "To Do" list was a joke. It wasn't going to happen because it was always put at the bottom of the list, and quite honestly, I wasn't even sure what I was supposed to be doing to relieve stress.

There is actually quite a bit of research that has been done and continues to be done throughout the world about stress and stress management. This complex interaction of brain and body, chemicals and neurons, is fascinating, complicated, and has generated many books dedicated to the neurological processes alone. But let's get down to the nitty gritty. What have stressed out researchers (who get stressed out figuring this stuff out for the rest of us) learned about reducing the stress and the toll it takes on our bodies and minds?

I have included common sense solutions backed by research to give you the most practical solutions. These ideas are not just more things to add to your to do list. These are practical, real solutions, not just one more thing to feel stressed out about not getting done.

The Six Burn Busters - Life Strategies to Eliminate Stress and Develop a Powerful Self-Care Plan

I am a YMCA girl at heart. The classic disco anthem, which extols the virtues of this international institution, stirs my soul and is pretty fun to dance to. I know every word. I went to summer day camp at the Y, took swim lessons and gymnastics class at the Y, and gave hundreds of volunteer hours to the Y, as a volunteer in the YMCA Teen Leaders' Club program. My concept of a fully functioning human being firmly resides in the YMCA concept of Spirit, Mind, and Body. That is, human beings have three distinct, separate, equally important parts of their being that must be fed, nurtured, and strengthened in order to live a healthy, whole life. In homage, the first three strategies I offer for stress management fit into these concepts I learned so long ago as a youth at the YMCA. The first three address WHO you are: a person with a spirit, mind, and body that can all be damaged by the effects of stress.

As a child, it seemed that if I wasn't at the Y, I was in church. I attended a lot of worship services. Besides my mother taking me to church every week for the usual Sunday visit, I also attended various churches and Jewish temple services with friends when I happened to be at their house when service times rolled around. Most kids would probably find a way to go home when their friend's mom yelled down the stairs, "Hey! We're leaving for church in 15 minutes! Be ready!" But not me. I actually LIKED going to church, and churches different from mine–all the better. So as you can imagine, I have heard a fair share of sermons in my lifetime. A phrase that I remember hearing many times is–how are you using your "Time, Talent, and Treasure"? There are as many ways to interpret those words as there are translations of the Bible (i.e., hundreds), but in relation to stress strategies, I think of them as *what* you do. Your time (how you spend it), your treasure (using your resources), and your talent (knowing yourself, using your gifts, and maximizing your potential) all make up how you spend your life. You can choose to spend your life in one of two ways: heaping more stress and tension upon yourself or creating calm in the storm that life brings. By developing a personal self-care plan that addresses all six areas, you can live a life that will help you stay centered, strong, and low stress.

WHO You Are: Spirit–Mind–Body

Spirit

I am thankful to live in such a diverse culture in the United States. Not only are there many beautiful skin tones and cultures of origin, there are many forms of faith and worship. I believe we are all as much spiritual beings as we are beings with a physical presence and a thinking mind. My personal belief is in a loving, personal God who says, *"I know what I'm doing. I have it all planned out–plans to take care of you, not abandon you, plans to give you the future you hope for" (Jeremiah 29:11; The Message).* In my most stressed times, even as I doubted myself, my calling, and all I believed in, I did not doubt that God would create a way out if I could just hang on. Granted, I wasn't always sure I could hang on. Somehow I always made it one more day. There have been times when I struggled to maintain spiritual focus and hope. Doubt and struggle are okay, giving up on your spiritual self is not.

As a busy woman, time to be quiet, meditate, pray, and seek seemed like a selfish luxury. Time for prayer and being with others who shared in my spiritual journey was something to be saved for when I had "more time." It was easy to put off till the next retreat or tragedy forced me to reflect. With a sense that God/church/spirituality will always be there, it is one of those things that can become easily neglected in the dedication of service to others. It is our spiritual selves that are most likely to become neglected as we give to others.

Spiritual health may be the most difficult piece of the puzzle for many of us because of the time and focused energy it takes to nurture within ourselves. It is also a place of deep wounding for those who have experienced abuse or bad counsel at the hands of spiritual leaders. Spiritual health cannot be faked or forced. Developing one's spiritual self is a personal ride that can be shared with others, but can only be started by the individual. It takes time and reflection to assess your own personal spiritual health, to know yourself in your spirit.

It is not necessary to be a "religious" person. In fact, I would caution against it. Rather, I suggest that you spend time getting to know yourself, your true authentic inner self. Your true self changes and is guided by what you connect with spiritually. This work is intense and meaningful if you allow it to be. Take the time to build that anchor for yourself. When you are left with yourself alone and the noise of the world or others fades away, your spiritual self is what remains.

Spiritual Self-Care

Long walks and sitting still – are these activities on your "to do" list? Are you constantly on the go? Always multi-tasking? Music on in the background everywhere you go? Should I stop talking about myself now? I know how it is. I am a multi-tasking mom myself, with too many irons in the fire, and I generally don't go anywhere without listening to music or talk radio. Trust me. I am talking to myself here, too, with the following admonishment. Practice the spiritual discipline of SILENCE. Take a walk or hike at the park by yourself, no headphones. Sit STILL. Sit in silence. Drive somewhere in silence and think, pray, and meditate. Sit and see if you can think, meditate, or pray for a full five minutes. If you have never sat in silence with yourself for five minutes, it might seem like an awfully long time. You can kneel and clasp your hands, sit cross-legged, strike a yoga pose or two, or just sit there. Being alone with your own thoughts can be a little scary at first. But you can do it, and the rewards are well worth it.

Develop your "inner life," where your ego (inner self) strength, simplicity, freedom, and truth can flourish (Wicks, 2006). Wicks suggests that one of the ways we develop this is through long walks, silence, and solitude. Every major religion and spiritual philosophy contains meditation and inner reflection as part of the path to enlightenment (spiritual understanding). This requires what some call spiritual discipline, but I call spiritual self-care. If loving yourself is the key to loving others, spend time alone, deeply knowing who you are, connecting to the deep inner strength you gain from yourself, God, the universe, others, whatever. Continue searching, growing, exploring, never giving up on that spiritual aspect of yourself and others. It will give you the insight you need to love yourself and, therefore, love others more deeply. Through that search, we gain the hope that we can and will connect deeply with others and ourselves.

Is it possible to find JOY in the burnout of hitting rock bottom? It's not exactly where people usually go to find joy and happiness. But what if that is the very place where you can refocus, connect deeply with yourself, and begin again? You may be reading this and are already at a point of burnout. Your joy has already been sucked out of your work, perhaps your entire life. Being in the place of burnout actually gives us the opportunity to find joy again. In *The Joy of Burnout*, Dr. Dina Glouberman recounts her own journey through burnout and recovery. She says radical healing is the shift that burnout asks us to make in our lives. It is as we surrender that the feeling of coming home begins (Glouberman, 2003). Powerfully, Dr. Glouberman offers this as a sort of meditation: "Before we burnt out, we gave ourselves away. Now we surrender to something larger than ourselves" (2003). When you find yourself in a place of burnout, be it mild or severe, consider it an opportunity. You will not get your life back. You will get a better life, an examined life. A life free of what you thought you needed–now focused on the important, vital things, and relationships.

Recovering from burnout is in many ways like recovering from addiction. Many of us come to a place of burnout because we are addicted to things like adrenaline, working, or proving how good we are. I've never really been addicted to anything unless you count carbs, Facebook, or getting certifications....well, um, never mind, but I am a devout student of the A&E network show *Intervention*. There is wisdom from the world of drug and alcohol recovery that applies to those of us who have become addicted to stress hormones, including adrenaline; multi-tasking/overwork; and saying yes. We need to take a look at the serenity prayer and take a page out of the 12 Step's *The Big Book* to learn how to seek a life of low stress living (12step. org, 2011).

The Serenity Prayer is short and sweet, and fits perfectly with the daily challenges a MBP faces:

> *God, grant me the serenity to accept the things I cannot change,*
>
> *Courage to change the things I can,*
>
> ***And wisdom to know the difference.***
>
> -Reinhold Niebuhr

The 12 Steps have been used since the 1930s to help individuals find freedom from negative behaviors. According to 12step.org, the steps are applicable to any addictive or dysfunctional behavior. I am not proposing that every MBP has a negative relationship to her work. For a small number of women, the term "birth junkie" is very real and the zeal for helping women consumes all else – marriage, children, and personal health.

Any behavior or set of behaviors that leads to a stressful breakdown or burnout could qualify as dysfunctional. It feels strange to label helping mothers and babies as dysfunctional, but when that help is delivered at the expense of your emotional and physical health or the health of your close relationships, perhaps it is dysfunctional enough to benefit from following all or part of the 12 steps in order to restore function and joy back to your life.

The 12 Steps

Step 1 - We admitted we were powerless over our addiction - that our lives had become unmanageable.

Step 2 - Came to believe that a Power greater than ourselves could restore us to sanity.

Step 3 - Made a decision to turn our will and our lives over to the care of God as we understood God.

Step 4 - Made a searching and fearless moral inventory of ourselves.

Step 5 - Admitted to God, to ourselves, and to another human being the exact nature of our wrongs.

Step 6 - Were entirely ready to have God remove all these defects of character.

Step 7 - Humbly asked God to remove our shortcomings.

Step 8 - Made a list of all persons we had harmed, and became willing to make amends to them all.

Step 9 - Made direct amends to such people wherever possible, except when to do so would injure them or others.

Step 10 - Continued to take personal inventory and when we were wrong promptly admitted it.

Step 11 - Sought through prayer and meditation to improve our conscious contact with God as we understood God, praying only for knowledge of God's will for us and the power to carry that out.

Step 12 - Having had a spiritual awakening as the result of these steps, we tried to carry this message to other addicts, and to practice these principles in all our affairs.

If this resonates with you, there are dozens of groups that use the 12 steps first developed for AA (Alcoholics Anonymous) or patterned after them. If you feel you would benefit from a program, visit http://www.12step.org for more information. For those of us who are susceptible to overwork, Workaholics Anonymous (WA; www.workaholics-anonymous.org) is a good place to find support and affirmation for setting boundaries. Online meetings and materials are available, along with traditional live meetings. If your stress or burnout has brought on additional problems, such as overeating or other addictions, support groups exist for nearly every addiction or behavioral challenge.

Basics of Spiritual Self-Care Strategies

- Spiritual exercise: long walks, sitting still, stretching/yoga. Do you take time to be alone in prayer and meditation while being conscious of your body?

- Times of silence. Do you spend time in quiet reflection?

- Moments of solitude. This can be at a place with other people, such as a coffee shop, but experienced alone, writing in a journal, doodling, thinking.

- Daily prayer time or time of gratitude/thanks. What great thing happened today that made you happy? Even if it was only one thing? What was it? Meditate on it.

- Think positive. Do you live for something larger than yourself? When the worst occurs, having a larger perspective can help you pull through until things are better. Consider keeping a gratitude journal to write life's triumphs and remember how you overcame the trials.

- Develop a serious hobby. Having a hobby–something that allows you to find joy in solitude (like painting or knitting) and that you can give your heart and soul to gives you purpose and meaning outside of the work you do. Take it seriously and schedule it on your calendar. Reward yourself with extra time when you have spent long hours working with clients.

- Are you in a time of burnout? Write down the lessons you are learning? What is important to you now? What activities, relationships, and things deserve your attention? Determine these things and honor your decisions about them by living accordingly.

- Explore the Serenity Prayer and 12 Steps. Take time to explore the principles of surrender that lead to freedom. If you have a problematic relationship with work, struggle with overwork, or suffer from worry, these tools may be helpful for you.

Mind

The human mind encompasses your personality, thought processes, knowledge, emotions, and attitude. Different from your heart or spirit, your mind is what might more accurately describe your soul or your thinking self. It is the seat of your thinking and understanding. As a Hypnobabies® Childbirth Hypnosis instructor, I educate my students about the conscious and subconscious parts of the mind. The conscious part of your mind is what you use to read this book, formulate your words, converse with others, and make decisions. Your subconscious mind is like an internal computer and contains all the memories, information, beliefs, and ideas that shape your conscious thoughts and actions (Tuschoff, 2009). You can address stress and burnout on conscious and subconscious levels to achieve calm, and even reverse the effects of stress.

Hypnosis can be used for stress management and addressing negative thoughts and behaviors. Hypnotherapy and self-hypnosis are powerful tools for making changes in your life, and they can be a regular stress relieving tool or centering activity. You may have the image of people on stage, clucking like a chicken; however, that is NOT the type of hypnosis I am suggesting. Deep meditation (a form of concentration) relaxation techniques, otherwise known as hypnosis, is a natural state. It is that same state of mind as when you stare off into space as you ride in a car or in an elevator, the last few moments before you drift off to sleep, or before you really consider yourself awake. It is something you do to yourself, for yourself. No pocket watch or magician is necessary.

How can hypnosis help you navigate stress? You can find recordings to download online or order custom CDs from hypnotherapists. They might be specifically related to issues you are facing, such as trauma, stress, or anxiety. Others might focus on being a confident doula, providing "sleeping peacefully" messages, or making healthier choices. Hypnosis is a powerful tool for filling your mind with positive thoughts and affirmations for a concentrated period of a time–on a regular basis for maximum effectiveness. Hypnosis and other therapies, such as brain mapping and EMDR, can be used to work through specific disturbing events, often faster than traditional cognitive behavioral therapy. A professional, licensed counselor can assist you with these therapies.

My favorite story concerning hypnosis is a story about my dear husband, KC. He had a trip for work to the high altitude city of Colorado Springs, CO, and shortly before leaving had been warned about how sick the change of altitude would make him. Co-workers warned, "Drink lots of water, don't do too much, and realize you will probably feel awful for the first day." Awesome. It wouldn't be a big deal for anyone else, but my dear hubby was a pretty severe hypochondriac at the time. Hearing that the altitude *could* make him feel bad was almost a sure prediction that he *would* feel bad. I suggested he get some hypnosis tracks for altitude sickness or anxiety, and he took my advice. As I checked in with him each day, he was drinking plenty of water, resting, AND listening to hypnosis recordings. Low and behold, each day he felt completely fine. Not a hint of altitude sickness! He was able to change a usual pattern of thinking, "If I can get sick, I will." to "Altitude sickness won't affect me." From weight loss to smoking cessation, resolving anxiety to birth without fear, hypnosis and positive affirmations are a powerful way to use your mind to improve your life.

There are other techniques for stress reduction and control that I refer to as "MBP mind tricks." If you know the Star Wars movies that serve as the cultural backdrop for anyone born after 1970, then you are familiar with Jedi mind tricks. If not, ask an eight-year-old boy (better yet, ask his father). Jedi warriors have "mind tricks" where they are able to make others think what they say. Mother-baby professionals can develop mind tricks that combat the negativity, guilt, and stress that can crowd our minds as we help struggling new moms, dads, and their babies. You aren't changing how others think; you are changing negative and stressful thought patterns in your own mind, as you choose any or all of these MBP mind tricks to put into place as a part of your self-care plan.

Using Your Work Switch

Switching On

It may help you to imagine a switch in your brain that you flip on when it is time to serve clients and flip off when it is time to leave them. Simply think of switching to your work self when you are on the way to a client's house or going into the office or work environment. Leave your "home self" behind. Leave the worries, concerns, and preoccupations of home behind; they can wait until after you are done. This allows you to give your full attention to your clients and focus on the task at hand. Having a singular focus will reduce feelings of being overwhelmed. Thinking about your home and personal life, while dealing with the needs of your clients at the same time, is the worst kind of multitasking. The truth of the matter is your personal problems will still be there when you are finished. Your client needs and deserves your undivided attention. You will utilize the information in your brain more effectively and be more in tune with your instincts if you are able to become YOU: the doula or YOU: the lactation consultant, instead of you – the stressed out mommy worried about your mortgage, kids, and bills, while also trying to focus on a mom with bleeding, cracked nipples.

Of course, you always carry with you the skills, wisdom, and courage amassed from your life experiences, but the goal of switching on to "work mode" is to focus on the task in front of you. The work of mother-baby professionals is so all consuming. You use your mind, intuition, emotions, and education, and maybe even ask for divine guidance to put all the puzzle pieces together and offer the support needed at that moment. When you give it all you've got, you will disable one of the guilt triggers so many of us suffer from. We feel guilty at work because we are thinking about our spouses or kids, and then feel guilty at home because we are thinking about work. Flipping that switch disables that trigger, so you have a singular focus instead of a divided mind and heart.

Many mother-baby professionals are self-employed. More hospitals are employing IBCLCs (or other breastfeeding support staff), and some childbirth educators, midwives, and doulas are part of hospital-based programs. Switching OFF is just as important to using this MBP mind trick as switching on. First of all, when you are self-employed, work never stops. You ARE your work. I know doulas that approach pregnant women at the grocery store or put their cards into baby related books at the bookstore. Besides those actions being questionable marketing tactics, they are also signs that the doulas are never turning off their "doula self" for fear of losing a marketing opportunity or reaching another mother. I want you to be a successful, relational marketer, but I also want you to know that you don't have to hand every pregnant belly you run into at the grocery store a business card. Put a magnet on your car and be done with it! It is not your job to reach every pregnant or parenting woman with the news of labor support or breastfeeding facts.

It can also be very difficult, self-employed or not, to set limits on your availability. Do you answer the phone AT ALL TIMES? It is better to have designated times when you answer the phone, send calls to voice mail, etc. Will you miss some potential clients? Maybe. But those who really need to contact you will leave a message or try again. There is a place of peace that comes from letting go of the obsession to answer every call. No one wants to feel they are leaving mothers without support or losing business, so "over communicate" with your clients. Include hours for phone availability on your voicemail. Include how long it might take to respond to email in your signature line or an auto email response. Give detailed voicemail instructions. For your peace of mind, do your best to let clients and potential clients who cannot contact you right away know how you intend to communicate with them and what they can do in the meantime. You can give special instructions to clients (like birth doula clients) whose calls you might need to answer immediately. Some doulas put clients' phone numbers in their contacts, so they know who is calling and can answer urgent calls. You can also change your voicemail to include the contact information for your back-up person or another community resource.

Secondly, it can be difficult to shake off the feelings and thoughts surrounding work with a client. Consciously switching off can allow you to "table" the challenges your client did or is dealing with, allowing you to give yourself fully to your home, family, and friends as you get back to the rest of your life. Switching off means you have given yourself fully to your clients and you can put that work down. There is a level of trust in our clients and trust in our interaction with clients needed to be able to switch off from work. The responsibility is yours to clearly communicate when and how your clients should follow-up with you; it is the responsibility of your client to contact you when they need or want to do so. My mantra is, "She's a big girl. She will call me when she needs me." If I start to get anxious that my client may need me, but might be reluctant to call, I call or email. If I don't hear back, I don't take it too personally. If I have done all I can to articulate how and when to call/email/text me and they have the resources to do so, then it is their responsibility to do it when they see fit. We have a tendency to think women in the perinatal period cannot be trusted to call on their support people. It is true that mothers do forget to call, get busy with the baby, or can be persuaded by others not to call, which is why a reasonable amount of checking in is okay. But it is also fine to leave some, if not most, of the responsibility with the client for continued interaction. Switching off from work makes you shake off the emotions and adrenaline produced during your service to mothers and babies, and refocuses you on your other commitments and joys. It will make the time with the ones you love sweeter and more focused, and make you more productive in your other tasks.

There is a popular gospel song that says, "Yes, after you've done all you can, you just stand." Just stand, knowing you've done the good work you know how to do, and without second-guessing yourself, put it away for a bit. Switching off keeps you from living in a permanent state of "what if." What if I had told her to do this? What if I had tried this breastfeeding tool? What if we had tried this pushing position? It is important to evaluate your performance from time to time, looking for ways to improve the services that you provide. That is very different from a constant feeling of "Did I do enough?" or "If only I could have thought of these things to try." Instead, think of every interaction with a client as an opportunity to grow and learn. Even if you are new to the field, having just finished your doula certification requirements or just passed the IBLCE exam (or another), you still have more knowledge and experience than your clients. You are never going to know everything. There will always be someone who knows more than you or who can see another perspective, or even help your client in a new and different way that produces more effective results than perhaps you can. On the other hand, you have a special set of personal experience, knowledge, and intuition that can help your clients in a way no one else can. You will be a different professional in five, ten, or 15 years than you are today IF you allow each experience to be a learning experience and not an exercise in how to beat yourself up. Just be you, do what you can, and *just stand*.

Basics of Switching Your "Work Switch" On and Off

Switching on:

- Have a ritual before beginning your work. Say a prayer, phrase, or a poem; listen to a specific type of music or artist; listen to positive affirmation; or read and repeat positive affirmations.

- Imagine a switch inside your body or mind, and visualize yourself switching it ON before meeting with clients. It's like flipping the switch to illuminate the OPEN sign at a place of business. You are mentally ready for the work ahead of you no matter how challenging.

- Before getting out of your car or walking into the room where your client is, close your eyes, take a deep breath, and say something positive to yourself, such as, "I am a wise, experienced IBCLC, and I will give excellent advice and support today." Open your eyes, exhale all the rest of your day/life away, and go in refreshed and ready to serve.

Switching off:

- Have a ritual at the end of your workday or time with clients. Make any notes of emails that need to be sent or things you need to have prepared for your next meeting, etc. Doing that ensures you will remember anything you need to do without having to actively hold it at the forefront of your mind. Leave your contact information with clients at the end of interactions (even if they have it somewhere else), and let them know how to get in touch with you. If it is a younger client who uses text messaging, and you do, too, you might even offer to text them at an appropriate time just to check in or remind them to call you for a follow up. (I know not everyone is comfortable with texting, but it is a major source of communication for those born post 1986.) Then say goodbye, close the file, and put it away until it is time to do follow up. Maybe you can listen to music. Sometimes it is good to have a different type of music than your "switching on music." Something happy, something reflective, or something uplifting. Experiment with a switching off soundtrack. Pray for your client or lift up a positive thought for them and their baby. Whatever is necessary to let the session/time go.

- Imagine your switch again, and remember to switch it OFF when you are done working with a client. This is a way to visualize making that mental switch from your MBP self to your personal self, and allows you to leave your client's burdens and hurts with them and fully give yourself back to your life and the people you love.

- After you leave your client, take a moment to close your eyes, take a deep breath, and say something positive to yourself like, "I offered caring, honest support to Elizabeth (mom's name) as she labored." That gives you something positive to take away from the experience.

- Listen to positive affirmations or hypnosis soon after working with a particularly draining client or in a stressful situation to restore positive thinking to your mind.

- Make notes or journal for a specific time (five to 10 minutes) to express any immediate feelings or thoughts, and revisit them later. This deposits your thoughts somewhere, so you can move on to other mind activities.

Slow Your Roll

Another MBP mind trick is to "slow your roll." My otherwise perfect children occasionally get a little too excited or get angry and lunge at a sibling. When that happens my husband, a former driver's ed instructor, says, "Slow your roll." Of course, the phrase comes from driving–you must learn to slow down or stop, and assess how to safely continue on the journey. In life, that means to SLOW down your emotions and reactions. I know you are excited/scared/angry/upset (or whatever emotion is spewing out of you), but calm down to a place where we can move forward. This is a mind trick you will most likely use during your work with clients. As you work with mothers and babies, there will be stressful situations. There will be situations that make you uncomfortable, anxious, sad, angry, and, of course, full of joy and exhilaration. It is easy to get caught up in the emotions your client is feeling if you aren't aware of its effect on you.

You will share in your clients' emotions. That is normal. It is healthy. It is part of the empathy we talked about earlier. It is a part of experiencing the full joy of humanity–sharing in the full range of emotions experienced during birth or postpartum service with moms. Taking time to *slow your roll*–taking stock of your feelings and thoughts–will help you focus, relax, and figure out your next move. Caring for your clients is an exercise in learning how to connect with them in a mentally healthy manner.

Recently, I sat with a young postpartum mother and her tiny new baby for a lactation consultation. As with many new moms dealing with breastfeeding challenges, she was emotional, teary, and fully feeling the intense love for her baby. She desired to feed her well, but was terrified it wasn't working. As she sat in my office, told me her story, and we worked together to get her baby feeding well, the weight of her emotions were palpable. I soon started to feel my emotions welling up. Her emotions and struggle took me back to the early days with my first newborn baby ten plus years ago. I so badly wanted to nurse my baby, and I wrote down every feeding and wet and dirty diaper for SIX weeks in order to make sure it was happening. I felt that deep, deep love she had for the tiny baby in her arms. The more I talked, I started to feel tears in my eyes. I felt like I was on the very edge of crying. Not that it is wrong to cry with clients. Sometimes it is 100% appropriate, but I knew I was going back to that place of being a desperately in love new mother.

I was able to slow my roll a bit and realize that I was getting more emotional than helpful to my client. I was feeling that I, to show her proper empathy and support, needed to pat her on the back, give her a hand squeeze, and help her develop a solid breastfeeding plan. It wasn't the time to be a friend to cry with. So, in that instance, I needed to slow it down a bit. I needed to slow my roll emotionally and empathetically, and let her know that it will get better and she can do it! In order to do that, I needed to pay attention to my own emotions and my own history, and how the two were interacting with my client's circumstances. I didn't cry with my client that day, and by the time she left, my emotions were down to a very manageable level. I wasn't worried about her or upset. I sent her off, giving her tools and knowing she would continue on the path that was right for her. For many MBPs, the emotions of clients keep them on a continual roller coaster. Slowing your roll is a tool that allows you to control the rollercoaster. You can give comfort and counsel without going on a ride with a client's emotions.

Basics to "Slow Your Roll" When Working With Clients

- Identify what you are feeling in relation to your clients' emotions. As they become upset, do you feel similar feelings rise up in you? This will not happen with every client. A specific experience, a specific client or type of client, or something else may trigger it.

- Explore the feelings you are having and allow yourself to determine how strongly you are feeling them. In order to continue supporting your client, do you need to slow your emotional reaction or continue with the emotional response going on in your heart/mind?

- Use techniques that can help you relax and calm down emotionally. Take some deep breaths, clench and release your hands, make a fist, and then shake and relax your hands, roll back your shoulders, or stretch. Sometimes doing something physical can "ground" you and help you take a step back from your client's emotions.

- Check in with yourself as you work with your clients. This is especially important when working with a client for several hours or in emotionally intense situations. Check in to see if you are maintaining a healthy distance. Offering understanding, non-judgmental support is key, but getting swept up in client emotions can seem overwhelming if you are not aware that they are influencing you. Getting swept up in their emotions can cause actions or words that are more like the support one might receive from a family member or close friend. If you are serving in a professional capacity, it is important to support the family to speak and act for themselves, accessing and exhibiting their own power.

- Check in with yourself after leaving a client. What is your mood? What emotions are you experiencing? Do they reflect any of the emotions you believe your clients were having during your time together? If so, ask yourself if they are really your feelings or if you have "adopted" them from your client. Take time to think about these feelings and talk about them with a trusted colleague, friend, or family member. Talking about it with someone may help you actually identify the feelings and whether or not they are your own.

What About Joy?

The following is a note about being influenced by joy. As mother-baby professionals, we, of course, are witness to moments of extreme joy, whether the birth of a child, a baby finally latching after weeks of not nursing, and many other amazing moments. MBPs often talk about being on a "birth high" or on a high from helping clients. The days I am able to get a previously non-latching baby to latch on and effectively transfer milk or to help a mother accomplish natural childbirth are much more likely to leave me feeling like I am great at what I do. If how I feel depends on whether or not my clients are happy when I leave them, I may set myself up for a lucky charm complex. Someone who focuses on themselves as the agent of their client's success or failure can lead to an inflated sense of self when things go according to plan and lead to feelings of guilt and shame when things don't. Should you be happy for your clients when they achieve their goals or share in their joy in becoming new parents? Yes, of course. I suggest, though, that your greater sense of joy comes from how you answer two things. Did I provide service and care that I can feel good about? Did I learn something from this experience that will help me serve clients better? If you can answer these two questions in a positive manner, you will experience joy beyond the moments of joy experienced with a client. You will experience joy from a job well done and a career that stimulates you and teaches you something new each day. This is a joy you can experience no matter what the circumstances.

There are other mind-based strategies that can help keep the stress that we feel as mother-baby professionals from overwhelming our lives. Checking in with yourself and others, giving yourself distance, and having a positive attitude are small but positive strategies that can change your stress levels for the better.

Checking In

First, let's talk about the process of checking in with yourself and others. Checking in with yourself involves taking a mental pause and evaluating how you feel. Am I feeling more highly stressed right now? Agitated? Confident? Concerned? It is about tuning into your feelings and seeing if you need more or less of something. Do I need a snack break? Am I thinking clearly? Am I feeling pressure to perform? If so, why? Checking in with others may take a while to establish as a regular habit. Checking in with yourself and others should help alleviate tension and stress, instead of feeling like just another responsibility. Think of it like a Facebook status update in real life. Share your feelings or thoughts and receive comments from your trusted colleague or friend. It could be a five minute conversation or much longer, whatever you need to take stock of what you are thinking and feeling. Checking in also connects you with another human being, banishing isolation. I often spend days working with clients and their babies, but have no interaction with my MBP peers. Checking in gives me that connection with others who are doing the same work and understand my frustrations and triumphs.

Checking in with someone does not have to be a formal process, but it may be best if you check in with another professional who shares your philosophy and ideas of appropriate care. This is someone you can trust with your thoughts and feelings and with any confidential information about a client you might need to include as you share your heart. Many who train together at a workshop (labor support or lactation related) stay in touch through message boards, online groups, or by exchanging phone numbers. Others may find each other through local networks, like a local birth network or lactation coalition. However the relationships develop, having one or two others you can trust and talk to regarding your work can make a huge impact on your stress levels. It is deeply therapeutic to be able to express your own disappointment about aspects of your work to someone who can understand. As much as our family members or lovers want to support us, they may not always understand where our deep passion and dedication comes from and how deeply we feel for our clients. Having someone to complain about the system with, strategize with, and even evaluate ourselves with is priceless.

Checking in with another MBP allows you to get thoughts you may have been thinking, but couldn't say get out of your head. Checking in gives you the opportunity to let emotions, confusion, and frustrations out, and may even help you recall things you would have forgotten without saying it, versus just living it once. It may or may not be a reciprocal relationship. I personally have a few close associates who I can share mother-baby related ups and downs with. It is a regular part of my work as a doula to call one of my doula practice team members shortly after attending a birth (sometimes on the way home) to discuss my concerns, stresses, and wonderful moments from the birth. I also make it a point to discuss lactation cases that leave me feeling "unsuccessful" with the other IBCLC in my practice. I am happy to lend a listening ear to other MBP friends who need to let things out after working with a client. It can be scary to open yourself up to another person, as there can be a lot of competition among professional women. Self-employed or otherwise, we all deal with concerns of being betrayed. Which is why checking in with others may be a piece of your self-care plan that takes longer than others. It involves finding the right person(s), developing a relationship, and then sharing yourself and your experiences. Until that is established, talking to a spouse or close friend may be your next best choice.

Giving Yourself Space

Giving yourself space is based on a tool suggested to therapists and helpers by Rothschild in *Help for the Helper* (2006). She suggests that therapists evaluate how their physical proximity to a client impacts how much they are impacted by the client's emotions. She asserts that maintaining a professional distance can help in creating firmer boundaries between self and client. Since the work of mother-baby professionals is so hands-on, creating a physical distance from our clients is not always possible or favorable. Sometimes small adjustments of physical or mental space can be made in order to give better care to our clients and create a healthier work situation for ourselves.

In the case of helping a mother during her birthing time, hands-on care, such as massage, letting the mother lean on you, or helping her get into position, are all part of the process. Much of the supportive work of labor is indeed in close proximity. As an experienced doula, I have noted that close physical contact is not always needed. It is okay and sometimes more beneficial to give a mother some space to be alone with her partner (if she has one), making it known that you are there if they desire your help or presence.

It can be helpful to just observe a mother in early birthing or during a time of change to clue in to her rhythms and rituals. Sometimes space is in the form of mental space. Mental space might mean reminding the mother that it is her baby and her birth, and you support anything she chooses to do (get an epidural, supplement with formula).

Heidi's experience with burnout illustrates how *giving yourself space* gives the choices and outcomes back to your client:

After a string of six clients who were induced, four of which ended in cesarean, I really thought I was completely failing at my job as a doula. I knew I had been educating them with the benefits and risks, but they were making extremely poor choices despite that. It took time (and perspective from colleagues) for me to realize that their choices (and the outcomes) were not my burden to carry.

Heidi Duncan, Birth Doula, Childbirth Educator, Perinatal
Fitness Educator

There may also be times that you have to remind yourself that no matter how hard you "want this" for a mom or "you know she can do it," you have to focus on the fact that this is her baby, her body, and her birth. She has made choices throughout pregnancy and birthing that have led to these moments. Let her experience be her experience. Your job as a support person is to give her accurate information, unconditional support, and loving reassurance. Things may not always go as planned; however, you can consistently give unwavering support that the mother will remember as feeling held up instead of alone. Whether mental or physical, giving yourself (and your client) space is another way to lessen the accumulation of emotional stress.

Basics of Giving Yourself Space

1. Evaluate the type of care you provide. Do you hover or feel the need to be hands-on, directing every move? Sometimes giving space can allow your client to try things without being dependent on you. You can end up giving her more confidence by letting her figure out something on her own. Taking a step back can also give you a moment to think, regroup, and come up with something new.

2. Take breaks for yourself. In birth work, it is important to take time to eat, drink, stretch, and even rest when possible. As a lactation consultant, going from patient to patient without so much as a granola bar will wear you down. Take time to take care of your basic needs, so you can give better care to your clients.

3. Take a mental step back. Remember this is her experience. Make it a point to ask your clients what their goals are and help them achieve them. Their outcomes are not necessarily a reflection of your care. A client getting a cesarean section doesn't make you a bad doula that didn't tell her enough or keep her upright enough, etc. Having a client whose baby doesn't gain enough weight one week doesn't make you a bad breastfeeding counselor. Remember the mantra – It's her body, her baby, her birth! Not yours.

It's All About the Attitude, Baby!

Stress research by Robert Sapolsky, Stanford University professor of biology and neurology, points to personality as a big influence on amounts of stress and stress-caused disease experienced by an individual. Sapolsky has identified five personality traits that influence stress levels and incidence of stress related disease that all have to do with personality or attitude. Is your personality a cause of stress? If so, can a conscious effort be made to change? I think so, but let's take a look at what the research has to say.

The five personality traits that influence stress level are:[3]

1. **Positive outlook:** Are you a glass half-full or a glass half-empty person? Do you see the silver lining or just the impending rainstorm? Do you see things as getting better or worse?

2. **Sense of control over your life:** Do you feel some control over your life or do you just wait for whatever is going to happen to come to you? Is there any sense of predictability?

3. **Perception of outcome of events:** Do you have a sense of whether or not the outcome of a situation is good or bad? In other words, can you recognize when you should still be upset about something or can you let it go when the time is right?

4. **What is your outlet?** Do you have an outlet for your frustrations or negative emotions?

5. **Social Support:** Are you socially isolated or do you have a group of friends you share life with?

You might already be putting together how these traits might affect one's stress level. I mean, it's not rocket science to understand that how you look at the world affects how you feel. When you look at challenging situations as opportunities instead of obstacles or choose to look at a disappointment as an opportunity to learn, the stress begins to dissipate. I have known some wonderful people who seem to do this effortlessly. They always seem to have a joyful, just-thankful-for-what-I-have attitude naturally. I, however, was not born with this gift. I have to work on it. I have to choke out the good attitude towards the half-full glass. I half jokingly refer to sarcasm as my true spiritual

---

3   For a very in-depth discussion on these and other factors that influence the effects of stress, see *Why Zebras Don't Get Ulcers: The Acclaimed Guide to Stress-Related Diseases and Coping* by Robert M Sapolsky. I cannot recommend it enough.

gift. I have to choose to see the positive possibilities, despite my default setting of sarcastic snarl. My true confession, though, is that when I give myself the gift of a silver lining attitude, things seem to go better. At least I am tuned in to the fact that things could indeed be worse. And it doesn't cost me anything to have a better outlook, just a change in emotional orientation.

I am a self-described nerd for all things pregnancy, birth, and lactation related. I will attend any lecture, workshop, or conference that I can get to, and I take related journals to the beach to read on vacation. So, when I was invited several years ago by a local CNM (certified nurse midwife) and university professor to have dinner with Henci Goer, esteemed pregnancy and birth author and speaker, I was thrilled and jumped at the opportunity. During the course of our lovely dinner, we talked about all things birth. I mostly asked questions and listened to her brilliant answers. Near the end of the evening, I asked a question, which I hoped, would bring an answer full of bright encouragement. I asked, "Do you think things are getting better (in the realm of birth and babies) or worse?" There isn't much that I remember clearly about that conversation other than talk about her newly born granddaughter and the answer to my question. Henci said almost immediately, "No." My heart sank a little. She went on to say that it wasn't getting better, not yet, but that wasn't the point. She then shared a well-known verse from the Talmud that has become a personal mantra and core belief for me. "It is not your responsibility to finish the work [of perfecting the world], but you are not free to desist from it either" (Pirkei Avot 2:16). It hit me like a cold winter wind after you've been inside for a few days, refreshing but a little hard to take. At first blush, it wasn't exactly the feel good answer I was looking for, but it was the truth. How can we say things are getting better with an ever-growing cesarean rate and inductions so common that the March of Dimes has to warn women not to ask for them? Maybe we can't point to massive, societal change at this point in time, but we can choose to be part of the groundswell. This generation may not experience the same cultural interest in natural childbirth and breastfeeding that advocates in the post-twilight sleep–pre-epidural era of American culture in the 70s experienced. But that doesn't mean it's time to give up.

We will have a new and different revolution. We can each choose to do our part, realizing that each of us, doing what we can, makes a difference. To remind yourself of how you help the individual mothers, babies, and families that cross your path, keep the thank you cards and pictures you receive from families in a special envelope or file. Print off thank you emails, pictures, and stories that mention your contribution. When you have a day when you wonder if what you are doing is really helping anyone (and they will come), pull out your file and go back through these notes. The impact on one life is incredibly important, as you never know the ripple affect your influence on that life may have. Know that you are somewhere in the chain, and your link is important, too. By choosing to have a positive outlook, you can actually impact your stress level for the better. If you think things are getting better, your stress hormones are lower and it actually makes things better. Feeling as if things are getting better helps keep the effects of stress at bay and gives meaning to your tasks big and small.

> *"To the world you may be just one person, but to one person you may be the world."*
>
> - Brandi Snyder

What about taking control? Do you hide in the corner, hoping to avoid a problem or do you take a deep breath and come out swinging? The research points in favor of meeting your challenges head on. Perhaps that relates to another factor in stress level discovered by Sapolsky's research that control or feeling of control and having predictive information both lower the effects of stress (2007b). When you tackle your stressors head on, be it difficult interactions with another person or getting over a fear like public speaking, you experience a level of control. At the very least, you are starting the interaction or experience. You have the satisfaction of getting things started instead of wondering when you might be surprised and forced to deal with an unpleasant situation. By taking control you establish your tone and actions. It may help you choose to be steady and calm, and control what you can. This can also apply to taking control of things like your schedule, your self-care, and your professional development. If you know you can only see two lactation clients a day and instead you schedule four because you can't say no, then you are not taking control. You are reacting to being asked for help by always saying yes. This can lead to stress and burnout from feeling out-of-control and overworked. If you never step away to eat or hydrate yourself at a birth, and then feel cranky, lightheaded, or weak during or after the birth, is it because you are reluctant to take control and take care of yourself? Are you concerned that you would upset your client? By taking control and taking breaks at well-timed, appropriate intervals, you can provide better care for a longer period of time. Taking control helps you make decisions that need to be made anyway in a proactive, rather than a reactive fashion. That little sense of control also lowers the effect of stress on your body, providing several positive effects.

Knowing whether the outcome is favorable to you is crucial in our somewhat counter-culture career field. As mother-baby professionals, we are sometimes in the position of being the odd one. We insist on things, such as skin-to-skin care and mother-directed pushing. These are some of the ideas we espouse that others we work with or beside think are crazy. A MBP can become so embattled and bitter that every interaction with a care provider is seen as negative and hostile. Do you see every medically trained person as the enemy? For example, when you are able to facilitate skin-to-skin care with a client, despite comments about the baby possibly getting cold (from the staff), do you see that as a victory or do you just see how they damaged the experience? By focusing on the positive of the events and seeing the victories small and large, you mediate the stress that can occur. In that situation, focus on the fact that baby got some skin-to-skin time. Maybe not as immediately or as long as you would have chosen, but you were still able to get your client what she desired and the baby what he/she needed. That is a victory, and if you choose to view it as such, it will help to decrease the effect of the stressful situation on you. When the outcome is not what you desire, take the time to evaluate the situation and learn from it. Then make sure you find a positive outlet for any negative emotions associated with the event.

An outlet for negative emotions is another key to reducing the affect of stress on your body and mind. We have discussed how important it is to have a hobby and to check in with someone else. Baboons get rid of their stress after a confrontation by taking it out on another weaker (lower) group member. Rats seem to suffer less stress if they can do something else when the stressor comes. Interestingly, it seems humans have similar behaviors. Perhaps I am the only mother who has yelled at my child when stressed because we are late, I can't find the car keys, and they still don't have a jacket on...but I think not. It is very common to take out our aggression that we cannot aim at the person or circumstances causing it on the people we love and have some authority over. We expect the person we love to forgive us, which can cause more careless behavior, including lashing out. The easy way here is not the best way. I tell my children that they may be angry, but they cannot hurt other people when they are angry. Life works a lot better when I walk the talk and follow that rule, too.

Develop a way to release your negative emotions, stress, and frustrations that doesn't hurt yourself or others. Scream out loud outside or into a pillow. Stomp, punch your bed or a pillow, or pour that energy into exercise (kickboxing, martial arts, and punching during dance style classes like Zumba® work wonders) or a long talk with your trusted professional buddy. Just know that releasing those emotions is a necessary step to lessening the effects of stress.

The single most important trait of the five is social affiliation or having friends (Sapolsky, 2007a). When looking at risk factors for disease, the most influential factor is poverty. The effects of poverty are such a significant stressor that it is a risk factor for disease and stress all on its own. Once we move past that, the next most influential factor is social isolation. After controlling for all other factors, lack of social connection contributes to a three-fold difference in mortality rates (Sapolsky, 2007a). Lack of community with others has a more negative effect than elevated cholesterol levels, smoking, and obesity on disease mortality rates. As human beings, we are intensely social animals. We need each other to survive. And as intense the need for a social group and friends are in teen years, the need continues to grow as we age. This protective effect of social connection is the same whether with a spouse, partner, group of friends, church family, etc.

Deep connections with others can actually save your life by keeping your stress levels low enough to avoid chronic stress related diseases or to provide people to help you realize when you are getting to a point of chronic stress and burnout. The exact mechanism isn't fully understood – all we know is that we need, really need, other people to survive and thrive. Relationships are not an optional part of life–they are essential. Are you spending time nurturing vital relationships? If you need to, put dates with your spouse, family, and friends on the calendar. Keep those dates just as strictly as you keep commitments to your clients. Relationships take time to build, so make the time. Take building personal relationships as seriously as making business relationships. It is the interactions with friends and family that will keep you grounded and sane during the most stressful times.

So what do you do if those personality traits don't describe you? Are you doomed to the ill effects of stress running rampant in your body and mind? I used to look at my personality, which consisted of the negative version of many of those traits and say, "it's just me. Get used to it. I'm sarcastic, I'm independent, and I don't have time for a hobby." Then when I started to understand the real importance of taking care of myself, my attitude began to change. When I realized that my stress level was directly impacted by my attitude, outlook, and how I decided to interact with the world, it became clear that not only could I change my "personality;" it was imperative that I do so.

Basics of a Burn-Busting Personality

1. Learn to put things into perspective. Learn to let the "little stuff" go, and learn to put more things in the "little stuff" category.

2. Be proactive. Take initiative when possible to give yourself some control over interaction with clients and others. Gather information to help you make decisions, but don't become obsessed with every detail. Control what you can and let go of what you can't. Remember the Serenity Prayer? Is your schedule out of control? Offer specific meeting times that work for you and stick with them. Do you worry about interaction with medical professionals? Introduce yourself and start the interaction off in a positive manner. Put your big girl panties on and take charge–you can do it!

3. Know the score. If all your work seems like a losing battle, you will feel like a loser. Is there something that can go in the WIN column for today? Was the outcome positive in some way? If not, proceed to the next item– your outlet for stress relief.

4. Let it out! Release! For many of us, bottling up our emotions, stress, and disappointments is a finely tuned skill. Unfortunately, this skill hurts us more than it helps us. Having an outlet or way of release will decrease the destruction stress can cause. Release can take many forms and be a regular activity or be specific to the type of stress. Regular release might include enjoyable exercise, play, prayer, meditation, listening to a specific type of music, singing, shouting, boxing/hitting a soft object, writing or blogging (perhaps anonymously), or anything else that is a release of tension for you.

5. Make a friend, be a friend. Regular, deep connection is essential to your humanness. If you do nothing else after reading this book, commit to forming deep vital relationships with at least three other human beings. They can be your spouse or partner, friends, or someone you would like to get to know better. As a social being, you need other people. Make it a priority to spend time being a friend–investing in the lives of others is a gift to you and to your friend. Schedule time to get together with others. Schedule dates with your beloved. Go out to lunch or out for coffee with that friend you haven't kept up with in a while. We all lead busy lives, but our relationships are what keep us going and help us heal emotionally and physically.

If you've been hurt and find it difficult to trust others, consider counseling, self-help books, or hypnosis to work through your trust issues. Healthy, deep relationships are not optional. They are vital to your well-being.

Body

Taking care of our physical self often takes a back seat to everything else in life. Have you ever visited a gym in the first two weeks of January? The place is packed with people who put themselves last all last year. It's impossible to get a treadmill! With the best of intentions to engage in regular sweaty activity, everyone in town has decided to make physical health a priority. There are all kinds of promises as the year begins, "It's time to take care of myself! I am going to go to the gym three days a week! I'll walk the treadmill, attend a class!" Then life takes over and we "run out of time," while still managing to get kids to activities, see clients, and do other life tasks. But somehow the priority of physical fitness often drops to the bottom of the list. Just check out how easy it is to get a treadmill in March!

I remember a conversation with my father in which I complained about not having enough time to do something. He corrected me and said years ago, "You have the time. We all have the same finite amount of time. The question is do you *make* the time for what you say is important?" We all have the same amount of time. Body related burn busters take dedicated time, which can seem like a sacrifice we can't give. It is difficult to take the time out each week to take care of our bodies, but there are strategies beyond the common recommendation to exercise for stress relief.

Body Awareness

Being aware of your physical reaction or arousal to clients or situations surrounding clients can help you reduce work related stress. By taking time to assess yourself, you can figure out when something starts to bother you and put into place steps to bring down your stress response. Do you hold tension in a specific place? Do you clench your jaw, have tight shoulders, or tighten your arm muscles when faced with stress? What about how your body feels during times of relaxation? Getting to know your body during relaxed times can also help you identify the differences that occur during stressful times.

Move Your Body – Sweat Is Your Body Crying Happy Tears!

Strength training and aerobic activity can help you burn fat and increase muscle, of course, but you can also think of it as building body armor. The concept of body armor as discussed by Rothschild in *Help for the Helper* suggests finding where you feel weak or affected when in stressful situations with clients and using strengthening exercises for those areas (Rothschild, 2006). It may help to specifically target areas where you hold stress or tension or "feel things" in a negative situation, or it may help to just know you are creating a stronger body all around. Muscles make you physically stronger, but there is also something about holding up your arm and seeing a rounded muscle or knowing you can walk or run a mile. You feel stronger as a person. You feel like you can conquer more.

Exercise can make you feel better inside, too. As little as 20 to 30 minutes of moderate exercise, two to three times a week has an antidepressant effect (Kendall-Tackett, 2010). Bending, twisting, punching, kicking, and dancing – anything that gets your heart pumping provides a release of endorphins– those "feel good" hormones. Exercise has the power to improve your mood as powerfully as anti-depressant drugs, and the side effects include better sleep and a better looking and feeling body. It may even provide the all important social support when done in a group setting (Kendall- Tackett, 2010). The exercise side effects sure sound much better than the side effects quickly listed at the end of anti-depressant medication commercials. So even if you don't consider yourself as a "fitness type," it's time to give physical activity a try.

During my deepest times of struggle I lovingly referred to Zumba® as my therapy. I did it every day – videos, classes, you name it. I probably needed that rush of endorphins more than I consciously knew. And after such a long time of putting myself at the bottom of the list, it felt really good to not let a day go by without doing something for myself for a few minutes. Part of my long-term plan has been not letting too many days go by without taking time to focus on movement and exercise. I schedule it on my calendar, setting an appointment for me and my body to spend some time together. It allows me to practice thankfulness! I am thankful to have legs, so I am going to use them! It's about appreciating myself and being the best I can be, not about being skinny or perfect. Finding a way to move your body in a way that appeals to you will give you a dose of customized hormones that can help pull you out of a funk. It's a great way to shake off bad feelings, a negative encounter with a colleague, or deal with frustrations. Even light or moderate exercise, such as yoga or Pilates, confer stress reduction health benefits, so make it a priority to find an exercise activity that can be your personal endorphin dispensary.

Feeling Sexy

Most MBPs are comfortable discussing things of a sexual nature as long as we are talking about clients. Most of us have seen more breasts or vaginas in one year than the average person does in a lifetime, but romance for a MBP is often one of those things that gets neglected. Why address this under body issues? Sex is a mind-body experience, especially for most women. Our minds and bodies have to be engaged for a fulfilling experience most of the time. Your body benefits in many ways from experiencing great, orgasmic sex, and you, as an adult human being, can and should experience that aspect of your humanity.

The research on sex is clear – it's GOOD for you (Cohen, 2010)! Women who have more sex have fewer menopause symptoms, lower blood pressure, and a lower risk of breast cancer. You burn calories every time you engage in the act and are more likely to have a healthy heart, too. It might not be worth it to just go through the motions; it seems orgasm or at least enjoying it is important, too. Besides all the wonderful effects of oxytocin and other happy hormones released during fulfillment, enjoyment of sex increases longevity for women. You are doing something for yourself and your body when you are enjoying a healthy sex life. Don't become a mother-baby eunuch because you are too busy or too tired for sex. Not only will it become a point of contention between you and your partner, it is missing out on one more thing that could be bringing you health benefits. Sexual healing isn't just a great R&B song by Marvin Gaye to get into the romantic mood; it turns out that sexual healing really is great medicine.

All Dressed Up and SOMEWHERE to Go

You may have heard the phrase, "the clothes make the man," but do the clothes make you feel better? Perhaps. Many professions, such as doctors, nurses, and law enforcement officers, among others, wear uniforms for many reasons, including easy identification to others. But what about how uniforms make the wearer feel? As a high school ROTC member, I can tell you that I felt pride in a clean, properly put together uniform. I am not suggesting that all mother-baby professionals wear uniforms or wear the same thing. The idea of standardizing what you wear might make you feel more powerful, polished, and professional. Your own personal uniform or standard dress can help you establish your work mode and your professional mode. Switching to your "work clothes" may help you flip that mental work switch to on and help your focus and energy while serving clients. Also, being able to change into other clothes after working with a client may help you move back to your private life.

Other variations of this concept include wearing a special piece of clothing or jewelry every time you work with clients. Some MBPs like to wear clothing that has a special birth or breastfeeding saying on it when working with families. There are many small companies that make beautiful necklaces, bracelets, and pins that symbolize pregnancy, birth, breastfeeding, mothers, and babies in a variety of ways. The jewelry itself holds no magical powers, but the symbolism you give it. If it helps you feel more grounded, secure, or comfortable, then it has all the magic it needs. Like having a lucky coin in your purse, some item of clothing or piece of jewelry that symbolizes to you what you do may give you comfort during stressful times.

Basics of Body Burn Busting Strategies

1. Build your body armor with exercise and/or weight training. I don't have to tell you all the reasons exercise is good for you! But you know now that it is just as powerful for your mind/emotions as it is for your physical health! Building strength in your body will make you feel emotionally stronger, too, so make time to fit in exercise and play!

2. Wear the right "power suit." Wear something that makes you feel strong, confident, and pulled together. If you look sloppy, you'll feel sloppy. If you look uncomfortable in your clothes, you will feel emotionally uncomfortable, too. Take time to find the right "work clothes" for you to feel your best.

3. Find your own Wonder Twin ring. Remember the Wonder Twins–the comic super heroes with a super ring that activated their powers? You might find that having a special shirt, bandana, scarf, or piece of jewelry makes you feel calm, grounded, centered, even peaceful, helping you think clearly during times of stress during work with clients.

4. Do some cardio. Cardio is very beneficial for stress reduction. The good news is stress relieving effects are observed with just 20-30 minutes of aerobic exercise a few (two to three) days a week. Regular exercise gives the most effective result (Sapolsky, 2004).

What You Do – Time, Treasure, and Talent

Time

Time is money.
Time is precious.
Time waits for no (wo)man.

We have so many sayings about time in modern culture. Clocks are everywhere–on our phones, in our cars, on our wrists! We are obsessed with how we spend our time, and we keep trying to find ways to divide and label our time as if it will create more of it. We read book after book attempting new strategies for maximizing it, managing it, and organizing it. But no matter what we do, there will always be 24 hours in a day. The sooner you (and I am talking to myself here, too) realize you have 24 hours and only you control how you spend it, the more you will be able to utilize your time in a way that brings you the most satisfaction and joy. Much of the feeling of "not enough time" that we as a society suffer from is a result of not valuing our time enough to do the things that we find really important. Instead, we do all the other things we think we can't say no to, and collapse at the end of another 24 hours just to do it again after a few hours of sleep.

Shame researcher and author, Brené Brown describes in her book *The Gifts of Imperfection* what I felt for so long and still struggle with today. "We've got so much to do and so little time that the idea of spending time doing anything unrelated to the to-do list actually creates stress" (Brown, 2010). She says we convince ourselves that those activities that would qualify as fun and play are a waste of precious time and that even sleep is for the lazy.

Think about your next 24 hours, your next year, five years, ten. What things are important long term? When you look back on your life, what will you want to have invested the precious resource of your time in? Spending time on yourself, your loved ones, and creating the things that no one can take from you (like memories) may end up ranking higher on your list than more work and accomplishments. If that's so–more relationships and memories on your life-long investment list – the question is: are you living in such a way that makes that a reality?

Sequencing

Young women and mothers today never imagined having to choose between raising children and having a career. We were raised with the images of Madonna and Claire Huxtable (never thought you'd see those two in the same sentence, huh?) as the modern women and mothers who had it all–all at the same time! What many of us have found is that the image doesn't always reflect the reality. Madonna ended up with a string of broken marriages and Claire Huxtable was just a talented actress reciting lines. The reality is that having it all, all at once, may not be all it's cracked up to be. If the stress of "doing it all" has taken a toll on you, consider the idea of sequencing your life goals and responsibilities.

Sequencing is the concept of having seasons of your life for professional work and seasons for focusing primarily on the home or self. For many women, this means pulling out of the work force completely for a season (usually to be at home with young children or a troubled teenager) to provide primary care for the home. It can also look like the period of time when you concentrate on getting an education for your future career choice while at home with young children.

Sequencing is also a concept that works at the beginning of a career. Interested in a career as a doula, midwife, or IBCLC, but have young children at home? A good place to start is by gaining knowledge. Put yourself to school. Read books, take online courses, join professional organizations, and attend conferences local to you. Shadow an experienced mother-baby professional or take a few to lunch and ask them about their challenges and triumphs. Why not be as educated and prepared as you can be before jumping in? You don't even need to be enrolled in a formal program or educational path to start your journey. You can even choose to begin your career with something more flexible and scheduled like teaching childbirth or breastfeeding classes or volunteering as a peer/community breastfeeding counselor.

Spending a period of time educating yourself and gaining experience takes patience when your passion to help is so strong and the need is so great. The stress load, however, is lowered when you can feel good about the time dedicated to home and family and are ready to shift some time and energy away to career. I think this is one of the primary reasons many younger women burn out of mother-baby work quickly. Faced with the intense needs of babies at home and the immediate needs of women in the perinatal period, the pressure becomes too much, and soon something has to go. Often women drop out all together, thinking it was just a phase of interest in the period of life they were in at the time. Those with a sequencing mentality, take time off from doing things that require them to be away from home/children for many irregular hours (such as primary labor doula work or on-call lactation work) and focus on community involvement, teaching, creative/craft work, volunteer work, reading, and blogging. Of course, you can overschedule yourself with any type of activity, so sequencing is also lived out by being mindful of how much time is being spent on what types of activities. Are you in a primarily working season or a primarily home season? And what does that look like for you in terms of hours spent in various activities each week.

The key to a season off of full-time or even part-time work is to continue stimulating your brain and keeping up your connections. Read blogs, articles, and professional journals in your field. Attend workshops, conferences, and keep certifications or licenses current. Even if you are not sure if you want to go back to your field, this keeps the door open.

At least once at every conference or workshop I attend, I meet a young mother with a toddler on her hip, a baby bump (she's expecting), and she is trying to get her certification finished, change the family diet to gluten free, and has a side business making scarves or something by hand. I remember being that ambitious, passionate young woman. I just couldn't wait to do it all with a baby on my back. I used to say, "Don't worry! You can do it! You'll get it all done!" Now I say, "You know, you don't have to do it all, NOW. It's okay if you take your time. Your children will only be little for a short period of time. Enjoy it; experience it. Being a mommy is the one job no one else can do." And usually I get a relieved look. It's as if someone finally can see that she just needs permission to put on the breaks and do one thing at a time.

So, here it is. I officially give you permission to give yourself permission to do what is right for you. That is the essence of sequencing. Saying NO to trying to do it all. That takes a lot of courage and faith in your destiny and ability to go against a culture that views exhaustion and productivity as badges of honor. It takes courage to say I can start and stop my "career" whenever I want. Trade in exhaustion and unrealistic levels of productivity for authenticity and courage as badges of honor. It will look a lot better on you, I promise.

Recovery Time

The time you spend in other activities outside of your passion has to be divided between responsibilities and recovery. Responsibilities are the things that have to get done, so no one goes hungry or naked. Recovery time is all that other stuff that needs to get done, so your soul isn't hungry or naked. As someone who fights for a cause each day, you need the recovery as much as you need the rest of it. Part of your job as a mother-baby professional is being an advocate. Our work often includes complex and stressful situations, including having to justify recommendations or helping a mother navigate the healthcare system. That takes a lot of compassion and patience. This type of work takes up a lot of mental and emotional energy. Taking care of your responsibilities insures that your basic human needs for food, shelter, and clothing are taken care of. Your recovery time is equally important, as it charges your batteries and gives you the focus for your responsibilities and passion.

You will still technically live if you are just doing the responsibilities, but you can only live that way for so long before your stress level begins to rise so high you can't see above it. Unfortunately, recovery time is often the first life ingredient to be canceled. Taking time for personal relaxation and "doing nothing" is seen as selfish or wasteful. What if it is actually one of the keys to being more productive and focused when you are doing all those other things you must do? If you are taking that time to relax and recharge, you will be able to give yourself more fully to your to-do list when it's time to focus.

What does recovery time mean? Recovery time is individual for every person, of course, but it can be put into practice in big and small ways, so it is always a part of your schedule. It is part of developing outlets to mediate stress. We talked about having an outlet as one of the five personality traits that help us conquer stress. Recovery time is your set aside time to develop those outlets.

You may already be thinking of things you can include in recovery time. Get ready for an extremely scientific suggestion–PLAY. Find ways to play and be creative. Seriously, you need play and creativity just as much or more than you need to be productive. I hope anyone that knows me isn't rolling his or her eyes right now. I am not always known for being the most playful person in the world, I admit it. But I really mean doing something purely for fun, to fool around, laugh, smile, and feel good! I know what some of you overachievers are thinking. I could run every day. Then I could get in my daily exercise at the same time. That's all WRONG! Stop thinking about how you can be more efficient! Nothing about this fun is efficient or involves multitasking. It is fun for the sake of fun and creativity for the sake of creativity! Now, if you love running or have always wanted to take it up, then it counts. For me, running would be about as much fun as cleaning base boards three hours a day, so I don't do that as my playtime. What does it for me is taking time to do things like reading magazines (non-academic), playing video games that include dance or movement, Zumba® classes, and hula hooping with exercise hoops. And don't let me find a dance floor, because there's never been one I didn't like. These are things I enjoy and can be done in a variety of locations with a variety of people. I am very social, so my recovery time often involves others. You might like more solitary time. Maybe you are more of a visual artist or perhaps you like to make things. Would you like to learn to play chess or get involved in Community Theater? Think of things you like to do or used to like doing. Is there a craft or class you have always wanted to take? Can you schedule a time tomorrow or in the next week to do one of those things for 15 minutes? (The answer is yes.) Put it on your calendar, do it. Repeat. Creativity and playfulness are a vital part of who we are. Take the time to embrace fun and creativity to give your soul time to recover from all the responsibilities and work in your life.

An end of the day, ritual is another recovery time activity. Many people struggle with falling asleep or staying asleep. It can be tough to wind down from a full day of helping others, especially mothers and babies who are in such a delicate time period. Think of the hour before you plan to go to bed as your time to prepare for sleep. Take time to get ready for bed, slow down your brain, and stop thinking about all the things you didn't get done today or have to do tomorrow.

One of my doula team members, Sarah McKay, keeps a note pad and pen beside her bed, so she can write down any last minute "I've got to do this tomorrow!" thoughts without having to get up. She says it helps her clear her mind and get ready for sleep. You can also write down one thing you are grateful for and something you are looking forward to the next day, each night before going to bed. Listening to affirmations or hypnosis before sleep is a powerful way to program your mind for positivity, so you wake up with that state of mind. And, of course, if it is something that appeals to you, a small glass of red wine before bed makes an excellent nightcap (or so I've heard). Rituals are a way of bringing order to our chaotic lives. Having an end of the day ritual might be the only order in your day, but it may be a small piece of relaxation and peace.

Basics of Time Burn Buster Strategies

1. Take some time (a few days if you can) to write down your ultimate life goals. What do you want to accomplish in your lifetime? What do you want to do professionally? As a parent? Spouse? Friend? Think about which of these goals are most important and at what point in your life you will need/want to focus on them.

2. Think about the season of life you are currently in. Do you have young children? Are you hoping to have children? What does parenthood (especially motherhood if a woman) look like to you in an authentic state? What other activities are important parts of your life? What can be put on hold?

3. Think, dream, and plan for your future. Sure, it can all end tomorrow, but plan for the next 40 years anyway. Going in and out of the workforce is commonplace today. Many people return to school later in life. The average person will have several careers in one lifetime. Plan your life in seasons or phases, knowing that you can focus on certain aspects at specific times. This sequencing can lower your stress level and relieve you of the superwoman/superman syndrome.

4. Make a list of things you like to do for pure enjoyment. Include small things, like reading a celebrity magazine, and big things, like taking a

cruise. Make a point to include these recovery activities in your life.

5. Develop an end-of-the-day ritual. It should consist of a few relaxing activities, such as a glass of red (heart healthy) wine, a cup of warm tea, a few moments of pleasure reading, listening to relaxing music, filing your nails, etc. Jot down a few notes before going to bed if anything is on your mind. You might have to write down your ritual at first to follow it. You can also just commit to doing something relaxing from a list of things you like each night. Once you know what you want to do, do your best to value yourself by doing it each night.

Treasure

In *The Joy of Burnout*, Dr. Dina Glouberman says, "We are in the habit of thinking that getting it done, whatever it is, is more important than how we feel. It matters; *we* don't matter" (Glouberman, 2003). We often value the things we do for others, thinking that is what they value in us. The treasure is what we are doing, the accomplishments we have, the "difference" we make. We spend all our time doing instead of being until burnout brings everything crashing in, and we can no longer get *it* done because we can't handle it any more. The first treasure you need is yourself. Recognize who you are—not what you do—as a treasure.

Giving Yourself Grace and Space

Giving yourself "grace & space" is the concept of valuing you, the helper, not just valuing the end product or the work you can produce. Living in Nashville, I know a lot of professional vocalists. Of course, there are those who party and live a reckless lifestyle, but thankfully, most of the ones I know take their craft and gift seriously. They know that their voice is a gift that has been honed by years of practice and training. Serious singers are aware that they have to take care of their throat, get enough rest, feel good, and have stamina for long performances and more to stay at the top of their game. They take care of their entire body, mind, and spirit just to sing well. They know bad performances can mean the end of a career. Service to mothers and babies requires you to take care of your whole self, too. Continually providing your service (your consultations and support instead of singing) without taking care of your instrument (your mind and body) can also end your career. Giving yourself "grace & space" is about valuing yourself as a human being, even if you can't get it all done. Value yourself, even if you have to tell people no or not participate in a project. Learn to honor yourself and believe that you matter even more than the work you produce. Without you, healthy and strong, your work will not continue.

Relationships

Treasure can also be found in the company we keep. Social affiliation or more plainly put, relationships, are a treasure no human being can thrive without. The movie *Cast Away* (released in 2000) was a moving illustration of the need for human connection. For the bulk of the movie, Tom Hanks' character was stranded on a tropical island with just a few items, including a picture of his girlfriend and a volleyball he decorates with a face and names Wilson. It might seem strange that a movie that primarily consists of a single actor would be about human connection, but the stranded man and his two objects reveal a lot about the treasure of human interaction and connectedness. Friends and family remind us of our past and our connections by re-telling stories of memories and helping build new ones. Therefore, the memory and hope of returning to his relationship with his girlfriend kept him connected to the world. But the companionship of Wilson, essentially an imaginary friend, kept him from losing his sanity. Fashioning a friend from an inanimate object gave him "someone" to talk to, and everyone needs someone to talk to. Wilson became his social network, fulfilling his sense of connection to another being.

Each person requires a different amount of "relationship treasure." You may be a more solitary individual or more of a "people person." I am not suggesting that we all should have tons of friends and keep in touch with all our extended family members. You can be lonely and have a lot of friends. I suggest that you reach down deep and focus on nurturing a few close relationships.

There are two types of relationships that are jewels in the relationship treasure box. The first is friendship and romantic relationships. It is likely that most of us will only have a few close relationships (and, of course, as many acquaintances and contacts as you desire). For many, those "close" relationships will consist of their spouse/partner and one to three friends. This is your inner circle. These are the people who you *know* and who *know* you. These are the people who you can be honest, authentic, and vulnerable with. They will love you, *the real you*, even when you can't give anything to anyone else.

Besides your romantic relationship, these close relationships may be people who share your passion, they may be friends, or they may be members of your family or faith. For some, an online community is a place to develop strong relationships. Online interactions through Twitter, message boards, online forums, and blogs, start on a surface level, but become deep as the interactions continue. Because you can seek those with similar interests (for example, a Yahoo group for private practice lactation consultants), you are able to find others who can offer you support and encouragement in a specifically stressful part of your life, but still provide interaction with people who have many differences (location, background, religious beliefs). Some projects, including social media campaigns, are run through online meetings and phone calls. Mother-baby professionals can work together worldwide without ever having face-to-face meetings. Attending conferences and workshops with online friends enhances online communication. For those who are hurt or disenfranchised from their local MBP community, finding an online community is a good way to begin to make connections again. It is also a good way to connect with others if there are not many MBPs in your area. Just a few years ago, internet-based relationships were not considered "real." Now it is common for people to identify close friends who they primarily developed a relationship with online. A mix of safe places online and IRL ("in real life") friends can make for a strong sense of social affiliation.

The second type of relationship treasure is the mentor. Mentorship treasure is when you have a relationship with someone older and/or more experienced than you who is willing to talk with you, answer your questions, calm you down when needed, or even be a shoulder to rant and cry on. Mentors help you keep this all in perspective. Mentors remember those feelings you have as a newbie and know what it feels like when the initial excitement wears off. Mentors understand the tightrope you walk between family needs and client needs. A great mentor will make time for you when you call and encourage you to do what is right for you, not necessarily what they did. Sometimes a mentor will just fall into your lap. You will naturally find someone, perhaps locally, in your field that can help you navigate your path. It can also be someone you meet at a conference or workshop who takes your calls and emails when you have questions. Others are blessed to participate in an apprentice model and are able to receive hands on, regular mentorship for a concentrated period of time. As you think about this concept, you may already have some informal mentors in your life. You may also be providing mentorship for someone else. The good thing about mentorship is that it is a treasure that gives to the giver and the receiver.

Gold – that's what most people think of when they hear the word treasure, right? So, I can't talk about treasure without talking about gold–or financial resources. It's clear that working in birth and breastfeeding is not a get rich quick (or even slowly) proposition. Just doing the work well requires a substantial financial investment. Education, training, buying supplies, marketing, and more are regular expenses from the beginning. Then there are professional organization membership, CERPs, and certification/licensing fees. The financial burden of doing what you love can be overwhelming.

Budgeting just a little of your payment for pampering or occasionally swapping services for something a client can offer is a good way to give yourself an extra bonus. Maybe consider a once a month massage or putting 10% of every payment you receive into an account to save for something special. Going to conferences is another way to use your financial resources reward from your work to enrich and restore yourself. Conferences are not just about gaining knowledge, they also include time for networking and countless opportunities to connect with others who share your passion.

Basics of Treasure Burn Buster Strategies

1. Give yourself "space & grace" by taking care of the instrument you use to do your work–YOU. Do you take time for yourself and supplies to eat and drink while working? If work is the reason you are eating fast food, becoming dehydrated, or drinking gallons of coffee, it's a possibility you are working in a way that does not make "space & grace" for you, the person doing the work.

2. Commit to modeling self-care, so you can teach it to your students/ clients. Be a role model. Commit to it for yourself, so you can teach it from a place of personal experience to your clients.

3. Social affiliation is measured in quality not quantity. Think about the people in your life you feel closest to. Has your work put your relationships with them on the back burner? Think about one to three relationships you can focus on. Spend the treasure of your time and emotions on those relationships by blocking special time for phone calls, emails, and get-togethers with them. Spreading yourself thin by being "good friends" with lots of people is more difficult than concentrating on developing deep relationships with just a few.

4. Do you have a mentor? Does someone come to mind when you hear that word? Have you ever told that person you look at them as a mentor? Let them know how much you appreciate their counsel and encouragement. If not, think about a person in your life who might be a good mentor for you. It doesn't have to be a formal arrangement, but it might help you to think about who fills that role in your life.

5. Budget a percentage or amount of mother baby related pay to an investment in YOU. From pampering to conferences to a night out with friends–using part of the money (even a small part) you earn to enrich and restore yourself is responsible and right.

Talent

Another interesting finding in the world of stress research is the impact of social rank on stress. Social rank or the amount of power you have to control your situation is important in combating the effects of stress (Sapolsky, 2007a, b). Those with more control or a better station have less stress. However, this is only applicable if the environment is stable. Leading in a community that is in constant turmoil (such as a country during a time of revolution) does nothing to help your level of stress; however, in a peaceful, stable community, having more power over your life brings greater calm (Sapolsky, 2007a).

How does this relate to your talent? Your talents are your gifts, the things you do well. Everyone can find something they are good at. Are you a good leader? Organizer? Encourager? Good at math? Words? Use those talents to lead others in some way. You can volunteer to be a committee chairman, help with a project, volunteer for a community organization, and/or seek to mentor or lead others professionally. By leading a group (even if small) or volunteering to help with a project, you can become the leader somewhere of something which, while bringing other responsibilities, may help you find a place of power in your life to balance the places where you do not have much control.

Another way to factor in social rank is to consider ways you might assume more control in your current work situation. Every day you help mothers learn to set boundaries and advocate for themselves as they care for their babies. Are you following the principles you teach mothers? Do you need to make changes so you feel like you are running your work instead of feeling like your work is running you? If you are working in a situation where you are not your own boss, find ways to assume more control of your work. Would you like to change some of the ways things are done? Do you have ideas that you think would be fun or helpful to implement? Just controlling some of the elements of your work situation may help you be happier and less stressed in your work environment. This may be even more of a challenge for the private practice professional. Setting limits that respect your time and the value of your services are key to helping you have more control. If you are self-employed, but feel the work never stops, perhaps that is because you never stop it. By putting limits on your work hours and communication with clients, you will be able to confine work to more specific times and places. This may at first seem impossible for mother-baby professionals, but in time you will see how you can set healthy boundaries and have more control over how your work intersects with your personal life.

Self-evaluation is a powerful tool for finding and developing your talents. You may not know what you are good at. Maybe you feel as if you used to be good at something, but now you're not so sure. You grow and change over time, even finding out new things about yourself. Even if you think you know exactly who you are and what your life goals are, it can be refreshing to see an explanation on paper. There are many personality profiles available in books and online to help you know and utilize your strengths. One of my favorites is StrengthsFinder 2.0 by Tom Rath. The Clifton StrengthsFinder (the assessment used in StrengthsFinder 2.0) has helped millions to "discover and develop their natural talents" (strengths.gallup.com). I found it to be easy to use and understand, with practical applications for life and work. Self-evaluation is not a one-time exercise. You may want to evaluate from time to time if you are using your talents to your fullest potential. Are you "walking in your gifting?" Are you doing work that maximizes your gifts and talents? Walking in your gifting is the process of consciously NOT trying to do it all. Do the things you are good at and that you enjoy, and learn to find solutions for the other things. Spending large amounts of time on things outside your areas of gifting will wear you down. Collaborate with others who have different gifts and talents, so you can share the workload. Trade services with someone who can help you with things you aren't good at, hire a professional, or find a way to streamline your more challenging tasks. Keep this in mind for both work and home life. You can maximize your gifting in the home. Are you a star in the kitchen, but hate doing yard work? Figure out how you can utilize the gifts (and preferences) of your household members, so everyone can pitch in and get the work done. Are your talents going untapped because you are stuck doing something that doesn't highlight the real you? Take the time to evaluate where you are and where your gifts manifest, so you can be your best and give your best.

Finding and participating in a local birth/breastfeeding/early parenting community is so important in order to use your treasure wisely. Connecting with others locally through discussion, social gatherings, political activism, community outreach, and just plain friendships brings opportunity for many of these stress-relieving strategies we have discussed. It also opens up opportunities for activism. Being involved in a local community may bring your attention to situations or people who can benefit from your expertise.

When you are well networked, you will know about opportunities to become involved with legislation, letter writing campaigns, and other ways to speak out. As Penny Simkin says, "The birth room is not the place for advocacy." And the time you spend with clients may not be the time to be in "fight the power mode," which can make you feel weak or ineffective. Carefully considering issues and situations in which you might stand up and speak out in a respectful, professional, but passionate way will be helpful for you to determine how much and what type of advocacy you would like to participate in. For some, writing letters, participating in protests, or just mentioning something in their email signature line or on their Facebook page makes them feel as if they are doing something to combat the injustice they see clients endure.

Being involved in a local community of mother-baby professionals also helps you stay connected to current information. You can't possibly attend every conference or workshop. You can, however, connect with others who may have gone. You can share and debate ideas, learn about new products and research, and hear about new books. Connection to your community of like-minded individuals, reading, and researching will make you stronger, smarter, and more well-rounded in what you do.

Basics of Talent Burn Buster Strategies

1. Become a leader. You don't have to manage a team of 50 doulas or a large lactation practice to lead. Lead in the community in a volunteer position or lead in something unrelated (coach your kid's basketball team, lead a book club, etc.). Lead for a short amount of time by offering to run a project with an end date, so you can see how it works out. Assume some control and leadership in some area of your life.

2. Find ways to assume control of your work. Do you feel like your work keeps you on the go all the time? Do you never get a break? Your work runs your life in part because you let it. Set boundaries, control more of when, where, and how you work to cut down on stress.

3. Do some type of self-evaluation test. StrengthsFinder 2.0 is available at bookstores, is affordable and easy to understand, and gives practical ideas on how to use the information gained.

4. Find a local community of mother-baby professionals and get to know them. A local community will enrich your life in many ways. If there is no local group (birth network, ILCA chapter, etc.) consider starting a local online group or getting one or two others together to start a group. This group can start as a simple encouragement group and grow into much more in a few years. This group can be a catalyst for many of the stress burn busters we have discussed.

It Comes Down to This

I'm pretty proud of you already for making it this far in the book. That means you are taking some steps to bring balance and peace to your life. Like I said earlier, I am not interested in adding more to your "to-do list." What all of this comes down to is whether or not you believe you are worth it. What you *do for* mothers and babies is worthy of praise and admiration. It is meaningful, impactful work. *But who you are matters more.* Because without you, without a whole and healthy you – your work will cease to contribute to our global tapestry of humanity. Your bright star will burn out and those tens or hundreds or thousands of moms and babies your work or influence impacts would be gone.

Through her work on shame, authenticity, and belonging, author and researcher Brené Brown discovered an essential truth that we all must realize in order to take the work of self-care seriously. In the *Gifts of Imperfection* (please promise me you will run, not walk to the nearest bookstore and buy this book next), she clearly draws the bottom line. She calls this type of living where you love and value yourself "wholeheartedness."

"Here's what is truly at the *heart* of Wholeheartedness: Worthy now. Not if. Not when. We are worthy of love and belonging *now*. Right this minute. As is" (Brown, 2010).

You need to start taking care of yourself now. Not after your next client delivers, not after you get through this busy season, not after you finish writing your curriculum. You need to care for yourself now, not once you have established your career, built your business, or achieved all your certifications. You are worthy of self-care NOW. Do you believe it? Say it out loud, right now. "I am worthy of love and self-care." Say it again, "I am worthy." Was it difficult to say? Even more difficult to believe? If so, keep saying it. Keep saying it until it is true for you. Because it comes down to this, if you don't believe that you are worth it, and that you matter more than the work you do, these suggestions and your personal care plan will just become more items on your "to do" list. You can choose to change your life and live from a new perspective that values you for who you are regardless of what you are accomplishing for others.

You are worthy. You are worth it. Believe it.

Chapter 6

Your Self-Care Plan

Keeping in mind these strategies, how do you develop a personal self-care plan that is right for you? In this section we will discuss assessment, plan, and life steps (APL). Your APL makes up your PSCP (personal self-care plan) and will change the way stress and burnout impacts your work and personal life.

The first step is assessment. You must first find out where you are. Are you already in a state of stress and depletion? Are you burned out? By first identifying what things are causing you stress and what things are off balance in your life, you can begin to see what needs to change.

Next, make your plan. Develop a philosophy of work, a way of life that works within your personal rhythm, allows you to be present, and honors you as much as your work. Decide how you will live instead of just letting life happen to you. Decide what you will say no to and plan to say it more often, so you can say YES to the things that really matter.

The final step is to walk in your life steps. It's all well and good to have a personal self-care plan, but it does you no good until you commit to living it. Put up reminders of your strategies. Let your family and close friends know how you intend to take care of yourself. Make a pact with a friend to check in on each other and make sure the plan is happening.

Of course, this is an ongoing process. This is not a one-time thing you can check off your "to do list." Thought about my needs, check. Nope, that's not how this works. You are changing your way of thinking, your attitude, and your path. Your personal self-care plan will impact all you do as you integrate it into your life. Some changes will be for a season; some permanent; and some will be daily changes. You will want to re-evaluate on a regular basis to make sure it is still working for you. Just as you are a work in progress, so are your stress relief techniques.

The following questions are meant to help guide you through the Assessment, Plan, and Life steps part of your PSCP. You will probably need additional paper, but may want to write short answers in the book or take notes. These questions are not meant to be completed in one sitting, but rather help you think and assess your current situation and develop a plan that you continue tweaking on a regular basis. Give yourself time, be patient with yourself, and let the answers come. They will.

Life Inventory

Home

Have you taken a personality or strengths assessment?

What were the results?

If not, make plans to take one. Which one do you plan to take?

Describe your home/personal situation:

What are your responsibilities at home?

What do you most enjoy about your home life?

What do you least enjoy about your home life?

Who are your most important relationships with?

I would like to add this to my home life:

If you could do ANYTHING in your personal life, your perfect fantasy, what would it be?

Why aren't you doing it?

What are your goals in regards to home/personal life?

The most stressful aspect of my home/personal life is:

My motivation for home is:

My vision for my home is:

My mission for my home is:

Work

Describe your job/work/career situation:

What are your responsibilities at work?

What do you most enjoy about your work life?

What do you least enjoy about your work life?

Who are your most important relationships with?

What are your goals in regards to work life?

I think I am fairly compensated for what I do: yes or no

Why?

If you could do ANYTHING in your work, what would your fantasy be?

Why aren't you doing it?

I would really like to add this to my work:

The most stressful aspect of my work is:

My motivation for work is:

My vision for my work is:

My mission for my work is:

Making My Personal Self-Care Plan

After answering the questions in the assessment portion, begin the strategies section. Look over all the Burn Buster strategies presented and pick those that may help you. Be prepared to visit this section often to review and change the plan. Choose at least one strategy for each area. Concentrate on your over-arching philosophy in that area and actual activities you want to implement.

Strategies:

1. Spirit

2. Mind

3. Body

4. Time

5. Treasures

6. Talent

Did you pick at least one strategy in each of the six areas? Write it down. Honor it. Live it. Share it with others.

My Personal Self-Care Plan

On a daily basis I will do these things to honor myself:

I suggest the strategies listed on the Pocket Helper Card available at http://www.proqol.org/Helper_Pocket_Card.html for 10 things to do each day.

I will take care of myself weekly through these activities:

Positive words I will use to describe myself:

I will treasure myself as much as the work I produce by:

When I am stressed I will take these positive actions:

After a difficult work experience I will:

My End-of-Day ritual:

Life Goals

(Personal, Family, Professional)

As you make your self-care plan, know that you are making a new path for yourself. This is the new super-professional path. If you want to help more moms and babies and change our world for the better, take care of yourself first, so you can be around for many years. If you want to serve your community, take care of your family and relationships first, so your home base is strong. If you want to be a bright shining star in the community of mother-baby professionals, don't let stress burn you! You are on the journey to a bright future with less stress and burnout may it be long, rewarding, and full of joy!

Epilogue My Story

I stared into the "vitamin cabinet" where we stored the vitamins, medicines, and such. It was early morning or late night–who knows–there comes a point when you've been up late so many nights in a row that it all blends together. Either way, I was the only one in the house still awake, and it had been that way for hours. Insomnia fueled by worry, stress, and bad dreams had kept me up again. Not to mention the research I had been doing on the very drug I found in the back of the cabinet. Thanks to the Internet, I could find out the side effects, but couldn't quite find the magical dose that would put me in the hospital, but not kill me. Just like I researched everything else, I wanted to make sure I did this just right. Negative thoughts overwhelmed me–my brain was on overdrive. All I could think about was this drug my husband had been prescribed for anxiety, but had elected not to take. Deciding it was too risky to take, he put it away in the back of the cabinet where it had stayed until that night when it called to me. And that night, my despair was so great that I was willing to do something desperate. I didn't want to kill myself. I knew the damage to my family would be too great. I was just desperate for a break, and the hospital seemed like a place where I could go. I shared the fantasy that many burned out, depressed women confess having–an accident that would land me in the hospital, but not kill me. It was as if an "accident" was the only legitimate way to get away. Just saying I needed a break would let too many people down, be an act of selfishness or weakness. I held the bottle in my hand not knowing what I was brave enough to do.

I turned on the faucet in the kitchen sink. I opened up the pill bottle, and in one motion dumped the pills down the drain. I was on the edge, but somehow dug deep and took a tiny step back. It was time to admit that despite the image I portrayed of "doing it all," somehow juggling family, successful self-employment, and more certifications than anyone I knew–the balls were dropping and I was spiraling out of control. All of the negative thoughts and emptiness were taking a toll. Spending every waking moment building a business, taking care of clients, and encouraging others had left me burned out like the underbrush in a California forest fire. I was at the end of myself. Ashamed, but too desperate to care, I knew "doing it all" wasn't working for me anymore.

Over the course of the next several months, I made radical changes. I stopped taking clients and teaching classes. I called a team meeting and informed my team members that I needed to step down, either closing the business or selling it. As much as I loved my business, I loved my life more. I figured if I had built up a business before, I could do it again. Several months later, we had a seamless transition from my leadership to another doula on our team. I took a break (not knowing if I would ever return) from all work–everything I had trained so hard for–and spent the next year reconnecting with myself and my family. I finally followed the advice I had given to struggling friends and clients and went to counseling for the first time in my life. I pulled the kids out of school to home school, took lots of field trips, spent time playing together, and made memories. I met with my nurse practitioner and began a plan to take care of my body, which was now suffering the toll of emotional stress, hormonal imbalances, weight gain, especially in my middle, and several deficiencies. I had to let go of keeping up appearances and do what I needed to do to save my family and myself.

Looking back, it's clear how things grew out of control. Our family had become broken by the weight of my drive to serve mothers and babies and create a career out of what I loved to do. As a mom, I had become completely disconnected. I was not emotionally or physically available. Answering emails, phone calls, and working with clients took up all my waking hours. Our oldest child bit her nails so severely she caused sores requiring antibiotics. Family meals–nutritious meals were a thing of the past. Weeks would pass with five nights being meals out because I had no time to prepare and cook meals. Several of us, including myself, had put on a significant amount of weight. I could feel myself becoming less healthy, more sedentary, and sluggish. And the marriage relationship, which had always been vibrant –full of laughter despite the challenges–was starting to feel optional. There were times when wedded bliss seemed like one more item on my list that I did not have time to check off. We swayed between trying to spend more time together and trying to avoid each other. There was never time to enjoy each other, only time to get things done in the brief moments we were together. Even when I was home, I wasn't home. And when I was gone, I could be at a birth for days only to be called away the next day for more work that demanded my attention. I foolishly thought if I could just work a million hours a week for a few sacrificial years, I would build something that would allow me to make money doing what I love. That's the American dream, right?

My dream was quickly becoming a nightmare. On the outside, I was the mother-baby professional who had it all together. In less than ten years, I had become certified by two doula organizations, held three lactation credentials, including IBCLC, achieved Hypnobabies® Childbirth instructor status, and had become certified or trained in a multitude of other mother-baby related titles. I was known around town and respected by families, members of the birthing/baby community, and care providers. Friend after friend would ask me how I did it all, which made me cringe every time. I wanted to tell them my dirty little secret. I'm not doing it. It just looks like that from the outside.

I would jokingly answer, "I live on the edge of insanity. Sometimes I drop more balls than I am juggling." Hoping they would catch just a little of my desperation. I knew it was all too much, but I couldn't say no to my own inner drive or to the needs of others.

Finally, after a series of work related crises and realization of the deteriorating family situation, I had reached a breaking point. I could no longer keep up the frantic pace of how I was conducting business. These critical events were the final snowflakes that toppled the avalanche. I refer to this time as a "mini nervous breakdown." In my mind, it didn't qualify as a true nervous breakdown (whatever that means) because it did not involve a straight jacket or sedatives, which is probably a terrible definition, but it made me feel a little better. I had always suggested counseling to others, but had never gone myself. I was understandably a little nervous. Being the "to do" list obsessed woman that I am, I just wanted to know two things: 1) Am I crazy? and 2) How long is it going to take to fix me? This "mini nervous breakdown" was messing with my life plan. I wanted to know if I was just having a momentary freak out or was I done with this career path. Did I just need to get a job at a retail store and move on? Was I going to be able to figure out how to manage my passion without it consuming me?

My therapist just encouraged me to be patient, let me talk through my initial issues and then go on to deal with deeper issues that had been the back-story of my life. Initially, my concern was, "Am I just not strong enough?" I thought perhaps I was a bad mother, a bad wife, a bad doula/childbirth educator/ lactation consultant, or maybe just an all around bad person. Maybe I was just selfish for wanting a career and having this passion. What I came to understand is that I had believed in my core that I was not lovable the way I was. I needed to do more, be more, and achieve more to be loved. My passion had been twisted into one more way to achieve, achieve, achieve in order to establish my worth. I had to be the perfect mother, perfect wife, and perfect mother-baby professional, or else NONE of it was good. My self-worth was directly tied to my ability to prove myself over and over. It was learning that I am lovable the way I am (totally NOT perfect) that opened the door for healing and freedom.

Since the "mini nervous breakdown" of 2009, I am not interested in how many balls I can juggle. When someone asks me, "How do you do it all?" I say, "I don't. I am trying to do less." It's still a struggle. As an obsessive multi-tasker and a driven over-achiever, I have to constantly focus on following my authenticity compass. Am I making decisions that will honor the needs of myself and those I love? Am I making a decision or a commitment that will help me reach my short and long-term goals? How will saying yes to this cause me to say no to something else? Recently, I began working with a business coach to keep me focused and low stressed. Talking with a coach each week keeps my actions in line with my goals, keeps me from saying yes to too many things, and reaffirms that I *need* to spend time on myself. I have learned to schedule less work and create margin for my life. I have learned needing sleep doesn't make me weak. I don't want the honor badge for being exhausted. I want to be able to have a long life with a loving family, doing the work I feel passionate about. I realize now that I can only do that if I pace myself, honor myself, and do less now in order to be able to do more in the long term.

I was able to slowly re-enter mother-baby work on a limited basis. Sequencing has become my way of work. I decided to work around my children's schedule as long as I see fit. By taking care of my physical and mental self, I can plan for a long life with many career turns and twists, starts and stops. If there is one thing we have as mother-baby professionals, it is job security. Women will keep having babies.

I currently take a very limited doula client load (maximum one to two a month, with some months intentionally empty) and teach Hypnobabies® Childbirth Hypnosis classes. I provide limited lactation services, seeing one to three clients a week. I take the month of December off, so I *never* miss Christmas with my family for someone else's family. My November and December teaching schedule is shared with another instructor, so we can both spend more time with family during the holidays. I read voraciously, keep up-to-date with research, and stay involved with social media. That helps me stay a part of the MBP community without hours and hours away from home. School field trips, kid parties, and Zumba® (hip shaking therapy) are unashamedly top priorities. Relationships with friends, a family of faith, my husband, and my personal needs come before all else. I have a renewed spiritual focus and I know that what I do each day has to honor who I am. If I spend my time neglecting myself and my family to teach others to nurture themselves and others, I will eventually be revealed as a fraud.

Each day I have to focus on loving and nurturing myself. It is a struggle to live in the now–to take time to do the fun and creative. It's hard to cut myself slack. When I remember that in the long run living a full, authentic life will actually make me better at what I do when I'm working, that me as a whole person is a gift to those I serve, I know I'm doing the right thing.

Stress continues to come, sometimes building again to what feels like a breaking point. Now, though, I know what my goals are and who I want to be. I have a plan for dealing with stress and burnout. I hope that as you have read through this book, you have begun to discover those things for yourself. Develop a personal care plan. Honor and treasure yourself. Mothers and babies need you to be healthy, so you can help them be healthy.

As you continue your journey of serving mothers and babies as you authentically nurture yourself, consider the words of funny man George Burns, born the ninth of 12 children, who worked until his death at age 100:

> *"If you ask what is the single most important key to longevity,*
> *I would have to say it is avoiding worry, stress, and tension.*
> *And if you didn't ask me, I'd still have to say it."*

Thanks for saying it George. Now here's to living it.

Resources and Recommended Reading

There are many wonderful books and websites that address stress and burnout. These are the resources I have found helpful. I would love to hear others that you have found helpful.

Books

Brown, B. (2010). *The gifts of imperfection: Let go of who you think you're supposed to be and embrace who you are.* Center City, Minnesota: Hazelden.

Glouberman, D. (2003). *The joy of burnout: How the end of the world can be a new beginning.* Makawao, Maui, HI: Inner Ocean Publishing, Inc.

Ilse, S. (1996). *Giving care, taking care: Support for helpers.* Maple Plain, MN: Wintergreen Press.

Kendall-Tackett, K. (2005). *The hidden feelings of motherhood* (2nd ed.). Amarillo, TX: Pharmasoft Publishing.

Sapolsky, R. (2004). *Why zebras don't get ulcers: The acclaimed guide to stress, stress related diseases and coping* (3rd ed.). New York, NY: St. Martin's Griffin.

Swenson, R. (2004). *Margin: Restoring emotional, physical, financial and time reserves to overloaded lives.* Colorado Springs, CO: Navpress.

Websites

General:

Helpguide.org - A non-profit website providing ad-free mental health information and encouragement.

Focusseminars.com - Focus Seminars of Kansas City Inc. is a professional organization that invites all to conquer life's challenges and move towards new levels of performance. Workshops guide you through the adventures necessary to gain a greater understanding of yourself and your relationships.

JanetFieldHypnotherapy.com - Clinical Hypnotherapist Janet Field offers customized guided imagery CDs, EFT Meridian Tapping, and more. She is also a Hypnobabies instructor and former doula and midwife and can understand the stress load of MBPs.

Ordinarycourage.com - A blog by researcher-storyteller Brené Brown, Ph.D. and her journey to live authentically and soulfully.

ProQOL.org - Information on compassion satisfaction, compassion fatigue, burnout, secondary traumatic stress, vicarious traumatization, and vicarious transformation. Includes The Helper Pocket Card with 10 useful daily strategies for stress reduction.

Birth Stress and Trauma:

Birthtraumaassociation.org.uk - An organization dedicating to helping people traumatized by childbirth.

Birthtraumacanada.org - An organization of mothers who have experienced negative childbirth experiences.

Solaceformothers.org - Solace For Mothers has a Yahoo Group for advocates and supporters of women with birth trauma.

Sheilakitzinger.com/BirthCrisis.htm - Website dedicated to help women who want to discuss traumatic birth. They offer reflective listening, not counseling.

Workshops for birth professionals who wish to do phone support are offered in her English home.

Tabs.org.nz - A Charitable Trust that supports mothers who have had stressful or traumatic births. Their goal is to make PTSD known as a form of mental illness that can happen following childbirth.

References

12Step.org. (2011). The 12 Steps. Retrieved on March 10, 2011, from http://www.12step.org/.

Antunes, S. (2009). Overcoming the three-year itch. *International Doula, 17*(2), 12-14.

Brown, B. (2010). *The gifts of imperfection: Let go of who you think you're supposed to be and embrace who you are.* Center City, Minnesota: Hazelden.

Cohen, E. (2010, January 7). New year's resolution: Have more sex. *CNN Health.* Retrieved from http://articles.cnn.com/2010-01-07/health/sex.health.benefits_1_health-benefits-sexual-activity-levels-of-stress-hormones?_s=PM:HEALTH.

Davis-Floyd, R.E. (1992). *Birth as an American rite of passage.* Berkeley: University of California Press.

Glouberman, D. (2003). *The joy of burnout: How the end of the world can be a new beginning.* Makawao, Maui, HI: Inner Ocean Publishing, Inc.

Grant, J., Lindstrom, K., Chamberlaine, A., Amram, N., Tomkinson, J., Rosinski, J., et al. (2010, August). *Celebrating commonalities of DONA doulas: Results of the DONA Pilot Study.* Presented at 2010 DONA Conference, Albuquerque, New Mexico.

Heinig, J. (2002). When the supporter needs support: Battling burnout among lactation professionals. *Journal of Human Lactation, 18*, 321-322.

Heinig, J. (2009). The dangers of the "do it all" mindset. *Journal of Human Lactation, 25*, 135- 136.

Kendall-Tackett, K. (2005). *The hidden feelings of motherhood.* (2nd ed.). Amarillo, TX: Pharmasoft Publishing.

Kendall-Tackett, K. (2010, December 1). Exercise as a treatment for depression in new mothers: It's as effective as medications. *Medications and More Newsletter.* Retrieved from http://www.uppitysciencechick.com/meds_more_exercise.pdf.

Lauwers, J., & Swisher, A. (2011). *Counseling the nursing mother: A lactation consultant's guide.* London, UK: Jones and Bartlett Publisher.

Larsen, D., Stamm, H., Davis, K. (2011). Telehealth for prevention and intervention of the negative effects of caregiving. Retrieved on March 14, 2011 from http://www.istss.org/publications/TS/Fall02/telehealth. htm.

Merriam-Webster's Medical Dictionary. Empathy. (2011). Retrieved on January 05, 2011, from Dictionary.com website: http://dictionary. reference.com/browse/empathy.

Proqol.org. (2011). *Professional quality of life elements, theory and measurement.* Retrieved on March 10, 2011, from www.proqol.org.

Rothschild, B. (2006). *Help for the helper: the psychophysiology of compassion fatigue and vicarious Trauma.* New York, NY: W.W. Norton & Company.

Sapolsky, R. (2011). Stress: Portrait of a killer. Retrieved on March 10, 2011, from http://killerstress.stanford.edu/.

Sapolsky, R. (Speaker). (2007a). *Stress and coping: What baboons can teach us.* (Audio podcast). Retrieved from the ITunes Health Library Stanford University – http://itunes.apple.com/itunes-u/health-library/.

Sapolsky, R. (Speaker). (2007b). *Why zebras don't get ulcers.* (Audio podcast). Retrieved from the ITunes Health Library Stanford University – http:// itunes.apple.com/itunes-u/health-library/.

Sapolsky, R. (2004). *Why zebras don't get ulcers.* (3rd ed.). New York, NY: St. Martin's Griffin.

Simkin, P. (2004). Doulas: Nurturing and protecting women's memories of their birth experiences. *International Journal of Childbirth Education, 19*(4), 16-19.

Simonds, W., Rothman, B.K., & Norman, B.M. (2006). *Laboring on: Birth in transition in the United States.* Routledge.

Smith, M., Jaffe-Gill, E., & Segal, J. (2010). *Understanding stress signs, symptoms, causes and effects.* Retrieved on March 10, 2011, from www. helpguide.org.

Solace for Mothers. (2011). *What is Birth Trauma?* Retrieved on March 10, 2011, from http://solaceformothers.org/what_birth_trauma.html.

Swenson, R. (2004). *Margin: Restoring emotional, physical, financial and time reserves to overloaded lives.* Colorado Springs, CO: Navpress.

Tabs.org.nz. (2011). *Could This Be PTSD?* Retrieved on March 10, 2011, from http://www.tabs.org.nz/diagnostic.htm.

The American Heritage® Stedman's Medical Dictionary. (2011). Empathy. Retrieved on January 05, 2011, from Dictionary.com website: http://dictionary.reference.com/browse/empathy.

Tuschoff, K. (2009). Hypnobabies® Childbirth Hypnosis for Childbirth instructor manual. Stanton, CA: Author.

Wicks, R. (2006). *Overcoming secondary stress in medical and nursing practice: A guide to professional resilience and personal well-being.* New York, NY: Oxford University Press, Inc.

Index

Author Bio

Micky Jones, BS, CLD, CD(DONA), HCHI, IBCLC, DFB

Micky's career began when she graduated with honors from Middle Tennessee State University with a degree in Consumer and Family Sciences, with emphasis in Child Development and Family Studies. She is a retired La Leche League Leader, Hypnobabies® Childbirth Hypnosis Instructor, Certified Labor Doula with DONA International and CAPPA, Hypnobabies® Certified Hypno-Doula, International Board Certified Lactation Consultant, Dancing For Birth Certified Instructor, DONA Approved Birth Doula Trainer, and perhaps most qualifying, the mother of three young children.

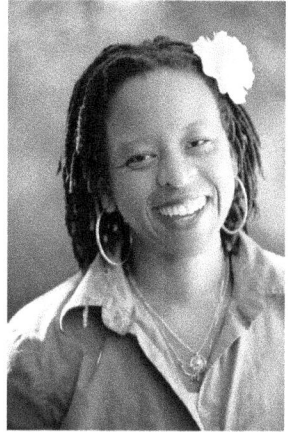

Micky's writings can be found in the blogosphere from time to time as a guest on various birth and baby related blogs. She can be found spreading baby related wisdom 140 characters at a time by following her on Twitter @ NashvilleBirth.

She loves to speak at conferences and train other professionals, and is currently focusing on developing workshop and conference presentations. She still works as an independent contractor with 9 Months & Beyond, LLC, teaching Hypnobabies® Childbirth Hypnosis classes, supporting women as a doula, and helping moms nurture their babies at the breast.

As part of her personal self-care plan, Micky explores play and creativity as a committed Zumba® enthusiast, hula-hoop diva, and occasional baker. She lives south of Nashville with her husband, KC, and their three children, Abigayle, Ambrose, and Paul.

www.ingramcontent.com/pod-product-compliance
Lightning Source LLC
Chambersburg PA
CBHW052038270326
41931CB00012B/2539